Issues in the Assessment of Bilinguals

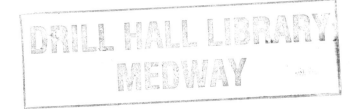

MIX
Paper from
responsible sources
FSC
www.fsc.org   FSC® C014540

Full details of all our publications can be found on http://www.multilingual-matters.com, or by writing to Multilingual Matters, St Nicholas House, 31–34 High Street, Bristol BS1 2AW, UK.

Issues in the Assessment of Bilinguals

Edited by
Virginia C. Mueller Gathercole

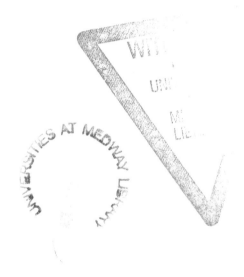

MULTILINGUAL MATTERS
Bristol • Buffalo • Toronto

Library of Congress Cataloging in Publication Data
Issues in the Assessment of Bilinguals/Edited by Virginia C. Mueller Gathercole.
Includes bibliographical references and index.
1. Language and languages–Ability testing. 2. Education, Bilingual. 3. Bilingualism.
4. Children–Language. I. Mueller-Gathercole, Virginia C. editor of compilation.
P53.4.I87 2013
404'.2–dc23 2013012133

British Library Cataloguing in Publication Data
A catalogue entry for this book is available from the British Library.

ISBN-13: 978-1-78309-009-9 (hbk)
ISBN-13: 978-1-78309-008-2 (pbk)

Multilingual Matters
UK: St Nicholas House, 31–34 High Street, Bristol BS1 2AW, UK.
USA: UTP, 2250 Military Road, Tonawanda, NY 14150, USA.
Canada: UTP, 5201 Dufferin Street, North York, Ontario M3H 5T8, Canada.

The policy of Multilingual Matters/Channel View Publications is to use papers that are natural, renewable and recyclable products, made from wood grown in sustainable forests. In the manufacturing process of our books, and to further support our policy, preference is given to printers that have FSC and PEFC Chain of Custody certification. The FSC and/or PEFC logos will appear on those books where full certification has been granted to the printer concerned.

Typeset by Techset Composition India (P) Ltd., Bangalore and Chennai, India.
Printed and bound in Great Britain by Short Run Press Ltd.

Contents

Contributors

Netta Abugov is a recent PhD student at Tel Aviv University and Marie Curie Post-doctoral Fellow at Tel Aviv University, Tel Aviv, Israel. Dr Abugov specializes in the acquisition and sociolinguistics of Yiddish in Israel and other Ultra-Orthodox centers.

Sharon Armon-Lotem is a Senior Lecturer at the Department of English and the Gonda Multidisciplinary Brain Research Center, Bar Ilan University, Ramat Gan, Israel. Dr Armon-Lotem's research focuses on typical and atypical language development in monolingual and bilingual children. She is the chair of COST Action IS0804 'Language Impairment in Multilingual Societies: Linguistic patterns and the Road to Assessment'.

Eli Arozena is a Research Assistant at the University of the Basque Country, UPV-EHU, Spain. Eli Arozena works on multilingual education in the Basque Country and Friesland in educational contexts where a minority language, the national language and English are used.

Rebecca Burns is an Assistant Professor at the College of Education, University of South Florida, Sarasota-Manatee, USA. She is the ESOL Coordinator in the College of Education at USFSM. Her research interests focus on the effects of linguistic knowledge on teacher performance and student outcomes.

Stephen J. Caldas is a Professor in the Doctoral Program in Educational Leadership at Manhattanville College in Purchase, New York, USA. His research interests include bilingual education and the sociodemographic correlates of educational achievement.

Jasone Cenoz is a Professor of Education at the University of the Basque Country, UPV-EHU, Spain. Professor Cenoz works on multilingualism and multilingual education by focusing on the development of communicative competence and the interaction between languages.

Shula Chiat is a Professor of Child Language at the Language & Communication Science Division, School of Health Sciences, City University London, UK. Professor Chiat has taught and carried out research in the field of speech and language therapy since the 1980s. The focus of her research is language processing in typically developing children and children with speech and language disorders.

Virginia C. Mueller Gathercole is a Professor of Linguistics in the Linguistics Program, Florida International University, Miami, FL, USA; and Professor of Psychology in the School of Psychology, Bangor University, Bangor, Wales, UK. Professor Gathercole has conducted research on monolingual and bilingual language acquisition in relation especially to semantics, morpho-syntax, and assessment. Her work also addresses issues concerning the relationship between language and cognition. She has specialized in Spanish-English and Welsh-English bilinguals.

Durk Gorter is a Research Professor at University of the Basque Country, UPV-EHU-Ikerbasque, Spain. Professor Gorter does research on multilingual education, minority languages and linguistic landscapes. He is the leader of the Donostia Research Group on Education and Multilingualism (DREAM).

Catrin O. Hughes is a Project Research Support Officer at the School of Psychology, Bangor University, Bangor, Wales, UK.

Emma K. Hughes is a PhD Student at the School of Psychology, Bangor University, Bangor, Wales, UK. Her PhD research focuses on bilingual aphasia, particularly cross-linguistic generalization of treatment effects in anomia.

Cristina Izura is a Lecturer at the Psychology Department, University of Swansea, Wales, UK. Dr. Izura is a trained cognitive psychologist interested in the cognitive and neural correlates of language in monolingual and multilingual speakers. She has published relevant work in relation to the order of word learning, dyslexia, word association, hemispheric differences in word recognition, Alzheimers patients, and lexical availability in L1 and L2 speakers.

Javier Marín is a Senior Lecturer at the Psychology Department, University of Murcia, Spain. Dr Marín is a psycholinguist mainly interested in the basis of visual word recognition, literacy, reading assessment, and dyslexia. He has also worked on L1 and L2 writing.

Theodoros Marinis is a Professor of Multilingualism & Language Impairment at the School of Psychology & Clinical Language Sciences, University of Reading, Reading, UK. Professor Marinis' research focuses on typical and atypical language development and processing in monolingual and bilingual children and second language learners.

Miguel A. Pérez is a Lecturer at the Psychology Department, University of Murcia, Spain. Dr Pérez has a Masters in Speech Therapy and a PhD in Experimental Psychology and has conducted research mainly on the neuro-cognitive basis of language in normal populations. He is currently focused on the influence of the order in which words are learned in first and second languages. He has also worked on the elaboration of psycholinguistic norms for words and pictures.

Rocío Pérez-Tattam is a Tutor of Spanish in the Department of Spanish, Swansea University, Wales, UK. Dr Pérez-Tattam's research interests concern the interaction between the knowledge of two languages in the bilingual mind, differential language development in bilinguals compared to mono-linguals, and issues of language assessment in bilinguals. She acted as a Postdoctoral Research Officer at the ESRC Centre for Research on Bilingualism in Theory and Practice, Bangor University, Wales, UK, from 2007 to 2012.

Kamila Polišenská is an Honorary Research Fellow at the Language & Communication Science Division, School of Health Sciences, City University London, UK. Dr Polišenská's research focuses on cross-linguistic aspects of typical and atypical language development. She is currently working on the development of clinical assessments for European lan-guages other than English.

Dorit Ravid is a Professor at the School of Education and the Depart-ment of Communications Disorders, Tel Aviv University, Tel Aviv, Israel. Professor Ravid is a linguist and psycholinguist working on the acqui-sition of language and literacy in typically developing and disordered populations.

Emily J. Roberts is a Project Research Support Officer at the School of Psychology, Bangor University, Bangor, Wales, UK.

Penny Roy is a Professor of Developmental Psychology, Language & Communication Science Division, School of Health Sciences, City University London, London, UK. Professor Roy's research focuses on early processing skills and language disorders, and the effects of early deprivation on language and literacy.

Belinda Seeff-Gabriel is a Clinical Tutor and Researcher at the Language & Communication Science Division, School of Health Sciences, City University London, London, UK. Dr Seeff-Gabriel's profile includes clinical practice, teaching and research. The focus of her research is the use of sen-tence repetition as a clinical tool when working with children who may have speech and language disorders.

Hans Stadthagen-González is an Assistant Professor of Psychology, University of Southern Mississippi-Gulf Coast, Long Beach, MS, USA. Dr Stadthagen-González is a psycholinguist with two main fields of interest: (1) Language interaction in bilinguals at the interface between morphology and syntax, and syntax and semantics and (2) Lexical processing in monolinguals and bilinguals, particularly concerning the variables that modulate word recognition and production. He worked as a Postdoctoral Project Researcher at the ESRC Centre for Research on Bilingualism in Theory and Practice, Bangor University, Wales, UK, from 2007 to 2012.

Enlli Môn Thomas is a Senior Lecturer in Education at the School of Education, Bangor University, Bangor, Wales, UK. Dr Thomas's main research interests span psycholinguistic studies of bilingual language acquisition, particularly in relation to children's acquisition of complex structures under conditions of minimal input, and educational approaches to language transmission, acquisition and use.

Feryal Yavas is a Senior Lecturer at the Linguistics Program, Florida International University, Miami, FL, USA. Dr Yavas's research and teaching interests include language acquisition (first, second and bilingual acquisition) and pragmatics/semantics.

Preface and Acknowledgments

The purpose of these volumes is to raise awareness of the issues involved in the assessment of bilingual children and adults, to suggest potential solutions, and to identify both theoretical and practical ways of approaching those issues in an informed, evidence-based manner. These volumes arise out of multiple links across the globe between researchers working with bilinguals from a variety of standpoints – theoreticians, clinicians, speech practitioners and educators. Many of these interactions were fostered in recent years by conferences sponsored by the ESRC Centre for Research on Bilingualism in Theory and Practice at Bangor University, its visiting researcher program, and other similar support.

Many people have assisted in various capacities in the preparation of this work. This includes participants at a workshop on the assessment of bilinguals at Gregynog, Wales, and the reviewers of these chapters, whose expert advice and insightful feedback helped to shape these works. In particular, beyond the authors of the chapters themselves (some of whom also acted in a reviewing capacity), I wish to thank the following reviewers and members of the Centre: Fraibet Aveledo, Isabelle Barriere, Dermot Bergin, Marketa Caravolas, Angela Fawcett, Tess Fitzpatrick, Bryn Jones, Rhonwen Jones, Manuela Julien, Debbie Mills, Simona Montanari, Betty Mousikou, María Carmen Parafita Couto, Ann Rivera, Seren Roberts, Kathryn Sharp, Elin Thordardottir and Mari Williams. Thank you also to an anonymous reviewer of the books here – your helpful comments and advice have served to strengthen and improve the volumes immensely. I am also very grateful to Kleanthes Grohmann for his generous help with technical computer issues.

A special thanks goes as well to Professor Margaret Deuchar, the Director of the Centre, whose wholehearted support, both moral and financial, has helped to ensure the success of this endeavor. I also wish to express my gratitude to Professor Colin Baker, whose unending encouragement for the volumes and the research in them is greatly appreciated, and to Dr James Sutton at FIU, who provided invaluable support in the final stages of preparation of these volumes.

A great debt of gratitude also is owed to the members of my research teams: First, my group in the Centre, who have been integral to the success of our work in the Centre over the last five years. Thank you to Rocío Pérez-Tattam, Hans Stadthagen-González, Enlli Môn Thomas and Kathryn Sharp. I also wish to thank researchers who have helped on several projects that have contributed to our work on assessment – in particular, Emma K. Hughes, Emily J. Roberts and Catrin O. Hughes, and two graduate students at FIU, Emily Byers and Erica Verde, who assisted in the preparation of the indices for the volumes.

I wish also to recognize the funding bodies who have helped to make this work possible. This work was supported in part by the following grants: ESRC and WAG/HEFCW RES-535-30-0061: ESRC Centre for Research on Bilingualism in Theory and Practice (2007–2012); Welsh Assembly Government: Standardized measures for the assessment of Welsh (2006-09), Continued development of standardized measures for the assessment of Welsh (2009-2012); ESRC RES-062-23-0175: Cognitive effects of bilingualism across the lifespan (2006-2012); and a conference grant from Gregynog, Wales. Without their support, none of this work would be possible.

Finally, the work here has profited greatly from discussions and collaborations arising from meetings of the Seminar Group 'Assessment of children from a bi- or multilingual context at risk for language impairment', headed by Carolyn Letts and Ghada Khattab, with members from all over the UK and from Europe, and funded by the ESRC Res-451-26-0707.

1 Assessment of Multi-tasking Wonders: Music, Olympics and Language

Virginia C. Mueller Gathercole

You don't get harmony when everybody sings the same note.
Doug Floyd (Guthrie, 2003: 41)

Imagine a world in which we saw beyond the lines that divide us, and celebrated our differences, instead of hiding from them.
Wesley Clark, speech, Jan. 20, 2004
(from http://www.notable-quotes.com/d/differences_quotes.html)

If a man does not keep pace with his companions, perhaps it is because he hears a different drummer. Let him step to the music which he hears, however measured or far away.
Henry David Thoreau
(from http://shell.cas.usf.edu/ ~ mccolm/Dquotes.html)

These volumes address an expanding area of interest and concern in the 21st century – the assessment of bilingual speakers, both adults and children. There is a rapidly growing body of research and proposals concerning the issues surrounding the evaluation of language abilities and proficiency in multilingual speakers, and, by extension, the evaluation of any cognitive or academic abilities in such speakers. Bilingual speakers' acquisition and knowledge of their two languages are necessarily different from acquisition and knowledge of a single language. This has ramifications for how bilingual speakers perform in a variety of tasks. If we wish to gain accurate evaluations of bilingual children's and adults' proficiency and abilities, we must necessarily take into account facts concerning the processes of learning, speaking, and understanding two languages. The authors in these volumes explore issues and solutions for the assessment of bilinguals. The research here comes from a variety of particular bilingual populations from around the world. The concerns expressed and the proposed solutions are relevant and applicable to bilingual populations everywhere.

Introduction

Some accomplishments in life are so remarkable that we glory in them and celebrate them. For example, we are in awe of people who show excellence in more than one aspect of a given talent at the same time. Some obvious examples come from the fields of music and athletics. We have great admiration for musicians such as Stevie Wonder, who not only wrote, produced, arranged and sang 'Superstition', but also played the drum, the clavinet, and the Moog bass synthesizer for it. We applaud the accomplishments of composers such as Georg Telleman, who played multiple instruments – violin, viola da gamba, recorder, flauto traverso, oboe, shawm, sackbut and double bass – and Paul McCartney, who plays the guitar, bass guitar, piano, harmonica, recorder, banjo, mandolin and drums.

We are equally awed by athletes that excel in not only one sport but two or three. Jackie Robinson, the first African American to play in major league baseball (for the Dodgers), had an illustrious career in baseball (e.g. winning the MVP award in 1949), but he also excelled in football, track and basketball while he was enrolled at UCLA (see http://www.toptenz.net/top-10-multi-sport-athletes.php#ixzz1rjaZWaIf). Jim Thorpe won gold medals in the pentathlon and the decathlon in the 1912 Olympics, and then he went on to play baseball for the New York Giants, the Brewers and the White Sox. He also played professional football and professional basketball (http://www.toptenz.net/top-10-multi-sport-athletes.php#ixzz1rjaZWaIf). We rightly applaud such multi-accomplishing individuals. It never crosses our minds that playing the drums in addition to the guitar might detract from the musician's accomplishments on the guitar, or that the athlete who excels in two sports might be inferior to someone who excels in only one of those sports.

We sometimes celebrate similar accomplishments in relation to language. We find it a surprise – but a delightful surprise – that Jodie Foster speaks fluent French in addition to English (http://www.youtube.com/watch?v=c3TvLSvvKMc&feature=player_embedded); that Salma Hayek speaks Spanish, Portuguese and Arabic; that Charlize Theron speaks Afrikaans natively (http://www.youtube.com/watch?v=2fYB9s0Nyzk&feature=player_embedded); that Natalie Portman speaks Hebrew (http://www.youtube.com/watch?v=n-PDArBZrz8&feature=player_embedded); that Sandra Bullock speaks fluent

German (http://www.youtube.com/watch?v=s10x38SMb-g&feature=player_embedded); and that Gwyneth Paltrow speaks Spanish fluently.

The majority of the world's population are just like these celebrities – they speak more than one language, and they often do so fluently. But somehow the delight and awe we experience in relation to celebrities who we discover are bilingual sometimes gets diminished or turned to caution in relation to others who are bilingual, especially in relation to children who are growing up bilingually. Why might this be? It probably boils down to two things: the important role that language plays in all aspects of our lives, combined with fear associated with a lack of knowledge about how bilingual language develops.

The way in which we view the multi-tasking accomplishments and evaluate the abilities of such multi-tasking persons hinges in large part on our appreciation of the steps one takes towards those accomplishments. Although we readily acknowledge those steps in the cases of musical and athletic advances, the steps in relation to language are perhaps more covert and less well understood. As we gain a fuller understanding of what it means to be a child growing up as a bilingual or an adult who has become bilingual, our understanding of how assessments of such individuals need to take those facts into consideration is also growing.

Step by Step

We tend to forget that people who end up being fluent bilinguals do not, of course, start out as fluent bilinguals – just as competent multi-instrumentalists or athletes who excel in multiple sports do not start life at the top of their art or their game. Everyone has to start from scratch. This means that budding musicians, athletes, and language learners all must go through multiple stages on the path towards coming to full mastery of their art. Those multiple stages involve multiple steps and periods when performance appears less than optimal. The emergent musician, athlete and language learner alike must, as a natural course of events, pass through moments at which errors are made and during which the prognosis for the ultimate success of the endeavor may seem uncertain.

To help the budding musician, athlete, or language learner and to gauge the level of his or her progress, we have ways of assessing whether that progress is commensurate with expectations, or whether, at points along the way, an emergent musician, athlete or language learner may need a little extra assistance along the way. There are exams and competitions children undergo in each of these realms, exams and competitions that entail expectations at a level that is determined by our knowledge of *how similar children or learners at similar stages of development have been able to perform*. Knowledge of that normal level of progress at each stage is determined by years, even centuries, of experience of observing thousands upon thousands of children passing through similar stages. For musicians, norms for such expectations are used in tests for performance at local, national, or international levels; for athletes, there are meets and competitions such as the Olympics; for language learners, there are tests of language abilities, especially in relation to reading and writing (and of related skills such as spelling), but also for oral language understanding, vocabulary knowledge and grammatical knowledge.

Tests related to musical and athletic prowess are usually not mandatory for every child passing through a certain age group or school level. Acquisition of these skills is seen as optional, and we tend to have the attitude that excellence in them involves specialist endeavors. So an inability to perform in either realm is not usually considered detrimental to a child's overall development, nor to have implications for any prognosis concerning their overall success in the future or as human beings.

With tests for language and language-related abilities (e.g. literacy), in contrast, the situation is quite different. All children are expected to achieve certain levels with language, and we take steps to assess their proficiency at multiple points in development. This universal testing of language occurs because of the fundamental nature of language as a key foundation on which success in a variety of areas that go well beyond language itself is built. Linguistic abilities are essential to academic success in all content areas, including not only those directly related to language (reading, writing), but also those that initially might appear to be independent of language, such as mathematical abilities. Unlike for musical talent or athletic abilities, therefore, there are high stakes associated with language abilities, as other successes appear contingent on a firm language base, which in turn is often taken as predictive of future potential in a variety of areas.

One consequence of this is that any evidence of possible difficulties with language are taken quite seriously by both parents and professionals, and any problems seem to be worthy of fairly prompt attention. For this reason, we assess children's language abilities very early on, and we continue to do so throughout a person's educational career. If a very young child does not appear to be talking when his or her peers are, a parent might take that child to a professional for consultation, to determine whether there are any major difficulties the child is having with language. When children enter school, they undergo tests related to reading readiness. Then throughout school, language and reading and writing assessments are key components of the assessment of a child's progress. Furthermore, when a child or adult begins to learn a language other than the first language, teachers administer tests to determine that person's progress in the second language.

Expectations

As noted, all of those assessments – whether for music, athletics, or language – involve underlying assumptions or evidence on realistic expectations for how a child or student should perform – *given his or her age, level, and experience*. For example, a 4-year-old Suzuki violin player might be credited with an excellent performance for being able to play 'Twinkle Twinkle' on his/her violin. No one would expect that 4-year-old to be able to play Brahms' violin concerto, nor consider that child deficient for not being able to do so. Similarly, a 4-year-old in a tumbling class might be rewarded with gold stars for making several somersaults in a row. Again, no one would expect that child to be able to perform a back flip like Aston Merrygold of JLS can.

In the area of language, a Kindergartner who is able to read at least a few words might be lavishly praised. No one would expect that Kindergartner to be able to read a text from Shakespeare or would test him or her on the understanding of a passage from *Hamlet*. (At the same time, if the same assessor or teacher is presented with a high school student who cannot read more than a few words, s/he might well be concerned and would consider whether such a student was in need of extra support.)

Children growing up as bilinguals

The realistic expectations we use to evaluate performance in any of these realms come from experiences with similar children or students at similar levels along the way toward gaining mastery of the skills. The present books are about what those realistic expectations might be for children growing up as bilinguals, and how we apply those realistic expectations in assessing performance. What might we expect at various stages in a bilingual child's or adult's progress in language? How can one tell whether a bilingual child is developing as might be expected, *given his or her age, level and experience* with the two languages, and how can we tell whether those expectations are or are not being met?

The educational and professional communities whose job it is to assess children's development have a good sense, and a long history of understanding, of how development occurs in monolingual children. The vast majority of the standardized tests for language have been developed with monolingual children or adults in mind (unless they are specifically designed to see if second-language learners have developed a command of their second language – e.g. the TOEFL (http://www.ets.org/toefl/). Typical examples are receptive vocabulary tests like the Peabody Picture Vocabulary Test (Dunn & Dunn, 2007) and the British Picture Vocabulary Scales (Dunn *et al.*, 1997). These provide information on the normal expectations one might have for monolingual children learning English in America or in the UK. (Note, however, that the BPVS now provides bilingual norms in addition to the monolingual norms.) Scales such as the Communicative Development Inventories (Fenson *et al.*, 2007) have largely culled data from a large number of (usually monolingual) children learning the given language to allow the assessment of other children learning the same language. And standardized college placement tests such as the SAT (http://sat.collegeboard.org/home?affiliate Id=nav&bannerId =h-satb) and the ACT (http://www.act.org/aap/) rely heavily on one's knowledge of the vocabulary and grammar of the language being tested, English. For example, the passage-based reading and sentence completion components on the SAT (see http://sat.collegeboard.org/practice/sat-practice-questions) require a knowledge of highly sophisticated vocabulary for accurate performance.

But we know that bilinguals' language development and their knowledge of their two languages is not the same as those of monolinguals (Cummins, 1981; Grosjean, 1982). This is because, first, bilingual children are hearing two languages, often in distinct social settings (e.g. maybe one language with grandparents, the other language at the preschool), and often with less cumulative exposure to each language than a monolingual child who speaks either language at the given age. At the same time bilingual children are experiencing some overlap in what they are learning about each language (e.g. learning two names for the same referent – *apple* and *manzana* – or two ways of talking about an action – *he ran away* and *salió*), and even some overlap of use in the same conversations, with code-switching common among bilinguals.

The unique ways in which bilingual or multilingual children experience language affects many aspects of development and the ultimate knowledge attained. This means that the timing of development can be different from that of monolinguals, that what they know in each language can be different and complementary (e.g. they might know the word for apples in one language, but not the other), that what they attend to may be different because of the 'packaging' of concepts in the two languages, and that their ultimate organization of the two languages will be different from the organization of either language in the respective monolinguals, with potential links between the two languages at multiple levels.

In addition, there can be important differences across bilingual children: Most importantly, the relative timing for when children begin each of their languages, or are exposed to each language (simultaneously from birth; beginning the second language a little later than the first, early in their preschool years; only beginning the second language on entry to school; or even beginning the second language later in life; and so on), matters for what course we might expect their language development to take. If both languages are developing simultaneously, the child's knowledge of the two languages may be relatively 'balanced', whereas if one language is begun after the first is already somewhat established, the latter may remain 'dominant' for some time, until the exposure to the second language has become more extensive.

Because language tests are designed to give some indication of whether a child is developing according to our expectations relative to a child's or speaker's *age, level and experience*, it is not really appropriate to apply a measure that was designed for one purpose (i.e. to gauge whether realistic expectations have been met for the course and timing of development in children who have been exposed to only one language) to use for a distinct purpose (i.e. to assess language development in children who have been exposed to two or more languages). This is true whether one simply wishes to know how well the child commands *this* language or one wishes to judge the child's overall linguistic abilities. In the former case, it would be uninstructive, for example, to use a measure designed for someone who has had, say, five years' experience learning the language with someone who has had only one or two years' experience.

But worse is the latter situation. When one wishes to determine, not only how much of language X a given child knows, but, more globally, whether a child is having particular difficulties with learning language *per se*, the importance of the language status of a child (monolingual vs bilingual) becomes heightened. Performing poorly on a second language (or on only one of a child's two languages) is not the same as having a systemic problem with learning language – just as the multi-instrumentalist's abilities in music cannot be totally gauged by only observing him or her playing the drums, or the athletic abilities of a child who has been playing baseball for four or five years and has just now begun track cannot be judged by observing his/her performance in track alone. To gain a full picture of a child's language abilities, the ideal would be to examine performance in both languages of the bilingual child to determine if there is a linguistic problem. If the child is performing up to expectations in one of the languages and not the other, that indicates that there is not a problem with learning language per se, just that the child is behind with a particular language. This is a critical distinction to make. An impairment that affects a child's abilities to learn language should affect both (or all) languages the child is trying to speak.

Goals of these Volumes

The chapters in these volumes attempt to tease apart some of the multi-faceted issues related to obtaining information on or determining the best ways of assessing bilingual children's and adults' abilities. The questions addressed include the following:

(a) What are the normal expectations regarding patterns of development in bilingual children?
(b) What are the normal expectations regarding ultimate linguistic abilities in bilingual populations and the roles of home language experience and community language in arriving at the mature command of the language?
(c) Is it important to assess both (all) of a child's languages?

(d) What is the best way to determine if a bilingual child has language impairment – LI or SLI?

(e) How does a professional assess language abilities in an individual if the assessor does not know the language(s) in question?

(f) How do we gauge development in a language for which no normed tests exist?

(g) Should tests be normed specifically for bilinguals?

(h) Are there potential universal means of assessing language abilities in bilinguals from distinct language populations?

(i) What effect is there on bilingual language acquisition when there is highly variable input?

(j) What sociolinguistic influences can affect bilingual language acquisition?

(k) How can we best deal with the assessment of language abilities in school children for whom the community or school language is an L2 or for children from a multitude of different language(s) spoken in the home?

(l) Are there strategies teachers can use to help improve students' acquisition of an early or later L2?

(m) Are there strategies teachers can use to build bridges between a child's home language and the language of instruction?

(n) What are the ultimate ramifications of educational policy on language instruction and on the use of the heritage language versus the school language?

These questions run through the chapters in the two volumes and are addressed from the perspective of the experiences of researchers and professionals working with a variety of populations around the world. This volume raises many of the ISSUES related to the assessment of bilinguals; volume 2 presents some SOLUTIONS.

Issues

Each of the chapters in this volume raises important issues that relate to assessment and constitute the basic motivation behind the search for any solutions that may be proposed for the assessment of bilinguals, addressed in volume 2, *Solutions for the Assessment of Bilinguals*. These underlying issues are at the heart of why improvements are needed in the forms and nature of assessments we apply to bilingual infants, children and adults – whether for the identification of language impairments; for children's progress, either in language or beyond language, in education; for L2-learners' abilities in childhood or adulthood; for general academic performance.

The issues raised in this volume are as follows.

(1) The first issue to be raised, in 'Why Assessment Needs to Take Exposure into Account: Vocabulary and Grammatical Abilities in Bilingual

Children', by Virginia C. Mueller Gathercole, Enlli Môn Thomas, Emily J. Roberts and Catrin Hughes, is as follows:

Issue 1: Normed assessments of language proficiency in children are in most cases normed on monolingually developing children. Such assessments, without norms specifically based on bilingually developing children, misrepresent the linguistic abilities of bilingual children. Assessments are needed that take into account bilingual children's level of exposure to the language in question.

Normed vocabulary and grammar tests are commonly used to assess children's language abilities, and, often by extension, conceptual abilities. Such assessments aim to determine whether a child is progressing in line with expectations, as determined by the performance of a large group of similar children, the norming sample. However, those samples often involve monolingual children, and the assumption that bilingual children develop in a similar fashion to monolingual children is unwarranted.

The normal course of development of vocabulary and grammar in bilingual children, and the influence of exposure are examined in relation to Welsh-English bilingual children aged 2 to 15. The chapter traces the effects of exposure on timing of development. The data support the position that initially timing of development is linked to amount of exposure, but that eventually, greater parity is achieved across groups.

Furthermore, the data are examined for evidence of crossover links, or carryover from one language to the other, especially in relation to grammatical knowledge. The authors examine children's performance on receptive tests of 13 types of grammatical structures in their two languages, Welsh and English. On the whole, the evidence is against carryover from one language to the other, at least on a linguistic level. Any links that can be observed appear to be attributable to links on another level, perhaps cognitive, perhaps meta-cognitive, perhaps meta-linguistic.

In addition, the ramifications for such data for assessment are discussed. The model followed by the *Prawf Geirfa Cymraeg* (Gathercole & Thomas, 2007; Gathercole *et al.*, in press) is advocated. In this model, bilingual children's performance is measured against two standards of comparison – first, relative to all children from their age range, and, second, relative to children from a similar home language background, with a similar level of exposure. Each child receives two standard scores under this model – the scores together provide a comprehensive picture of the child's abilities in relation both to the language in question and in relation to legitimate expectations, given the child's level of exposure to the language.

(2) A second issue is addressed in 'Assessment of Language Abilities in Sequential Bilingual Children: The Potential of Sentence Imitation Tasks', by Shula Chiat, Sharon Armon-Lotem, Theodoros Marinis, Kamila Polišenská,

Penny Roy and Belinda Seeff-Gabriel. The issue they raise is as follows:

Issue 2: Given the patterns of development in bilingual children, how is it possible for speech therapists to assess language abilities and identify language impairments or language deficits in bilingual children? This is an especially intractable issue when assessments are not available in the child's L1 (and when, often, the assessor does not speak that L1).

Given that bilingual children's abilities develop at a distinct pace from those of monolingual children, one cannot simply use tests designed for monolingual children to determine the language abilities (or deficits) of children who speak an L2. Low performance by the bilingual child in the L2 may reflect limited exposure to the L2, not a developmental deficit. So what is needed is some way of testing children that can reveal language *abilities* but does not require that the child have extensive exposure to the language being tested.

The ideal might be to test children in their L1. But this is not always possible: In today's context of mass migration around the world, there are increasing numbers of children whose home languages do not match the language of their (adopted) community, and increasing numbers of L1 language backgrounds represented among those children. (A recent survey of speech and language therapists in one borough of London, for example, found that during one month of 2011, therapists treated children who spoke 67 different languages (Shah, 2011).) In this context, it is next to impossible to develop batteries of tests to cover every pair of languages that are represented among the bilingual children. So the question is whether there is a way for professionals to test such children on their L2, the community language, and be able to distinguish the language-impaired children from those who simply have not yet had adequate exposure to the L2 to perform well.

Chiat *et al.* explore one alternative, the possibility of developing a language-neutral assessment measure. They examine specifically the possibility of using a sentence repetition task, in the L2, to act as such a measure. The authors point out that it has been shown that performance on non-word repetition tasks is subject to knowledge of the target language in question, but they explore whether sentence-imitation tasks might be more impervious to such effects.

The authors report on the performance of four groups of bilingual children of immigrants in three countries, speaking Russian-Hebrew or English-Hebrew in Israel, Russian-German in Germany, and Turkish-English in the UK, on sentence-imitation tasks in their developing L2 (here, Hebrew, German, and English, respectively). They compare the children's performance with monolingual norms, and also examine the extent to which age of onset (AoO) of the L2, length of exposure to the L2 (LoE), socioeconomic (SES) level and the structure of the test itself play roles in affecting performance.

The results show that, indeed, a majority of bilingual children performed within the monolingual ranges for the tests. At the same time, the data show that a substantial number fell below that range. AoO seems to play a role in performance: Those who begin the L2 before age 2 in particular perform similarly to monolinguals, but at later AoO ages, other factors seem to affect how similar the L2 children perform relative to monolinguals. SES plays a role, in that at least for some of the data, children from lower SES levels are more represented in the low-performing groups than those from higher SES levels; LoE seems perhaps less influential; and structure of the test itself is significant.

The authors propose that such sentence imitation tasks show some promise and are worthy of further research. The tasks are clearly helpful in determining children's *proficiency* in the L2, but they may also prove eventually to be a valid means, at least in some settings, of singling out children with language impairment. As these authors suggest, the effectiveness and usefulness of the procedure await verification through evidence from further testing.

(3)   In the following chapter, 'Assessing Yiddish Plurals in Acquisition: Impacts of Bilingualism', Netta Abugov and Dorit Ravid address the challenge of the assessment of bilingual children's performance in their L1 when that L1 is highly variable and is under continuing influence from the dominant language in the larger community. The issue they address can be formulated as follows:

Issue 3: Does one need to take into consideration the fluidity of language patterns in a bilingual community to assess bilingual children's acquisition of complex morpho-syntax in the language(s) they are learning? Most assessment measures rely on there being an established norm for each given structural element being assessed, and the test examines whether a child has reached that norm. But what happens when the morpho-syntactic element being examined is in flux, undergoing changes even in the adult language? How can we assess a child's accomplishments in regard to that element?

In this chapter, the language of interest is Hasidic Yiddish spoken in Israel, used in a context in which the language is in a fluid environment in which there is widespread contact between Yiddish and Hebrew. These researchers examine the use of plural marking, a highly complex system, on words in this dialect of Yiddish. They first elicit the forms for referents from adult speakers of the language, and they find that adults show a high level of variation in the forms they use for each word. Almost half the words take two or more plural forms, some words taking as many as four forms or more. These plurals have evolved in a sociolinguistic setting in which new Germanic-based forms, as well as Hebrew and Loshn-Koydesh forms, have evolved. These researchers then elicited 60 of these forms from children aged 3 to 17. These children's plural forms are highly consistent with the choices in the adult language, but they also show overextensions, some revealing influence from the contact language, Hebrew.

Such data raise the question of the best way of responding to the language of bilingual children growing up in a context of highly variable linguistic input and sociolinguistically fluid environment. How should one evaluate and assess their performance? What phenomena should be considered acceptable, as following the norm? Such questions are important, since bilingual children in such a contact situation across the world are often 'penalized', or their abilities are underestimated, because the forms they use do not reflect those of the standard norm. While children's variable choices can be seen to eventually parallel those of the adults around them, in terms of the proportions of usage of the available forms for a particular lemma, how should children's responses at earlier ages be construed? If younger children's performance is in line with the general choices available in the language, even if not entirely consistent with the patterns for the particular given lemma, should this perhaps be taken as positive evidence of children's sensitivity to the range of options available in the language they are learning?

(4) In the following chapter 'Measuring Grammatical Knowledge and Abilities in Bilinguals: Implications for Assessment and Testing', Rocío Pérez-Tattam, Virginia C. Mueller Gathercole, Feryal Yavas and Hans Stadthagen-González address an issue concerning assessment of bilingual adults:

Issue 4: Simultaneous and early bilinguals may differ in subtle ways from their monolingual counterparts on their knowledge and performance on each of their two languages. Assessments of grammatical abilities often take for granted that L2 learners may well differ from native speakers in performance, but little attention is given to whether speakers who are bilingual from birth or early in life may also differ in performance in subtle ways from their monolingual peers.

These authors explore the use of a receptive grammar measure similar to that used by Gathercole *et al.* (this volume), for Welsh-English children, with Spanish-English bilingual adults. The adults represent a population whose acquisition of their two languages can be considered to have occurred in optimal conditions – they are highly educated and grew up in an extensively bilingual community, Miami. They either were born and grew up in Miami or immigrated to the US as children and grew up as L1 Spanish-L2 English speakers in Miami; all grew up in homes in which mostly Spanish was spoken (OSH) or both Spanish and English (ESH) were spoken. These bilinguals provide an optimal picture of the grammatical proficiency in each of the two languages of a bilingual at the end-state.

As in the study of the Welsh-English bilinguals, 13 types of structures were tested in parallel tests for Spanish and English. The tests reveal a number of results. First, all of the bilinguals, regardless of group, performed equivalently in English. That is, no matter what the initial exposure to English in the home, all groups end up as adults with parity in their understanding of the English structures tested.

With regard to Spanish, however, there are differences across the groups. First, among the bilinguals, those who grew up in homes where both English and Spanish were spoken performed below those who were L1S-L2E bilinguals. There are also some interesting differences across the groups by structure. In one case, there is evidence that the monolingual Spanish speakers pay greater attention to an important Spanish-specific morphological marker than those who come from OSH and ESH homes. The marker in question is the object marker *a*, used specifically in relation to animate direct objects, as in *Juan la/le quería a María* 'Juan loved Maria' (cf. *Juan quería helado* 'Juan wanted ice cream'). In other cases, there is some indication that the bilingual speakers may be carrying over a distinction in English that is less relevant to Spanish. One of these involves the comparative versus the superlative: The bilingual speakers appear to make a more definitive demarcation between these for Spanish *más ADJECTIVE* versus *(el) más ADJECTIVE* than monolingual Spanish speakers do, possibly because of the clear distinction in English between the comparative and superlative in English. These effects suggest that, while the bilinguals on the whole perform very highly in Spanish, there are some distinctions in their processing of items that differ in subtle ways in the two languages.

In addition, even though all of the participants were themselves college students or graduates, there were differences in their backgrounds as children. When performance is examined relative to mothers' and fathers' education and professions, the performance on English was consistent across groups, but for Spanish, those from higher SES levels, as judged by fathers' professions, performed better. These results are consistent with those of Stadthagen-González *et al.* (this volume), among others (see also Gathercole & Thomas, 2009). They differ somewhat, however, from the results of the previous chapter showing that children's developing abilities in their two grammars are not on the whole related. This, along with the results of Stadthagen-González *et al.*, suggests that the linking of commonalities between a bilingual's two languages is more an emergent property of their knowledge than a developmental property.

(5)   In another chapter, 'Assessment of Bilinguals' Performance in Lexical Tasks Using Reaction Times', Miguel Á. Pérez, Cristina Izura, Hans Stadthagen-González and Javier Marín raise an issue with regard to assessing the total range of knowledge in a bilingual:

Issue 5: If assessments of bilinguals' language abilities aim to pinpoint exactly where their performance is similar to and differs from that of monolinguals, sometimes behavioral performance on vocabulary and morpho-syntax may not be enough. Performance on such tasks may mask underlying differences in the processing of language by bilinguals and monolinguals. Most assessments of bilinguals rely exclusively on such behavioral responses, so they do not capture fully the bilinguals' abilities.

These authors suggest that researchers should consider employing reaction time (RT) measures, so far uncommon in standardized tests, to assess language abilities in applied settings. Reaction times constitute a well-developed assessment measure used in cognitive and psycholinguistic research, and these could easily be adapted for use in evaluating bilingual performance. These authors use reaction time measures to assess L2 learners' acquisition of new vocabulary items, with special attention to whether assessments reveal important information on the efficiency with which learners acquire 'early' words (i.e. among the first to be learned) vs. 'later' words (learned after an earlier store of L2 words has been acquired). That is, they explore whether assessments accurately reveal order of acquisition effects.

These researchers provide a useful overview of the uses to which RT measures are put in experimental psycholinguistic studies, with special reference to their use in tasks of three types – lexical decision tasks, categorization tasks (including go-no-go tasks), and naming tasks (both picture naming and word naming/reading). They propose that because of advances in technology and the availability of resources, it is now possible to consider the benefits of bringing RT measures more directly into applied assessment settings.

They demonstrate the contributions that RT measures can make with a study examining the effect of order of acquisition (OoA) on processing and acquisition of words. OoA is a measure purported to be related to the relative timing or age at which words were acquired – e.g. *bread* might be acquired at age 2, whereas *earthworm* might be acquired much later, maybe after age 5 or so. Theories have been developed concerning whether words learned early are acquired, processed, or remembered more easily than those learned later. In a study in which these authors trained monolingual Spanish speakers on words from an unfamiliar language (here, Welsh), they examine the accuracy and RTs of learners according to the OoA of the given words. Although their results reveal no difference on *accuracy* for the early versus later words, RT data reveal *subtle differences in performance* on the early versus late words. Those subtle differences provide evidence on the ease of learning and retaining words learned early versus those learned later. These authors argue that such effects can be exploited by those wishing to develop more sophisticated or more subtle measures of bilinguals' and L2 learners' abilities with language.

(6) In the following chapter, 'Assessment and Instruction in Multilingual Classrooms', Rebecca Burns turns to the classroom and issues related to assessment and instruction in a multilingual classroom:

Issue 6: How can teachers assess and instruct multilingual students in their classrooms when they themselves have no knowledge of the first language(s) of their students, and when assessments usually take place in the students' L2? Not only does this lead to an underestimation of the child's knowledge, but it misses a prime opportunity to use the L1 to enrich the acquisition of the L2 and bridge the cognitive gap between learning through the L1 and the L2.

Burns raises this important issue for educators. As multilingual students and students limited in proficiency in the L2 used in the classroom become more and more the norm in our ever-shrinking world, the question of how the teacher might make use of the student's L1 for instruction and assessment becomes critical. As Burns points out, studies have shown that young learners have greater academic success when the school they attend shows an appreciation for diversity. Most importantly, teachers' use of the L1 of the child in assessments and teaching serves to support, rather than detract from, the acquisition of the L2 as well as to provide a bridge for the transfer of cognitive knowledge in academic domains.

The author takes a very practical approach and provides some useful guides for teachers on how to both assess and support children who are L2 English learners (ELL children) in their classrooms. Her suggestions revolve around the language resources increasingly available on the internet from around the world. She demonstrates how the teacher can draw on the L1 to boost literacy skills, to bridge between the L1 and the L2, to assess those skills, to provide content instruction (including translations), and to assess content knowledge. She provides something of a 'cook book' of tips for teachers, and she provides a useful compendium of resources on the internet that can be helpful in many ways to teachers. Some of these resources can provide translations, some materials in other languages, some information on the aural pronunciation of other languages, and so forth. In short, she argues and shows that the L1 can be the teacher's ally in the L2 child's education and evaluations of progress.

(7) The following chapter, by Jasone Cenoz, Eli Arozena and Durk Gorter, 'Assessing Multilingual Students' Writing Skills in Basque, Spanish and English', continues the investigation of assessment in education. They address the following issue:

Issue 7: How do children fare in contexts in which bilingual education is the norm, and children are exposed to a third language, in each of their languages? Does it matter whether children are taught through the medium of the minority language of the community vs the majority language? What level of proficiency do they arrive at in each language? And what is the evidence on academic achievement under these conditions?

These authors address these questions by examining patterns of performance by Basque-Spanish bilingual children in the Basque country. The authors provide a lucid overview of types of bilingual education programs throughout the world, and follow with a detailed description of those available in the Basque country. Three educational models are followed there, and parents have a choice of which model they wish their children to attend. In *A model programs*, Spanish is the language of instruction and Basque is studied as a second language. In *B model programs*, both Basque and Spanish are languages of instruction, each for approximately 50% of school time. Basque is also studied as a second language in this model. In *D model programs*, Basque is the language of instruction and Spanish is a school subject. In addition, although several languages are options to study as a compulsory foreign language, English is increasingly chosen.

Cenoz *et al.* review the evidence, first, on the academic performance of children growing up in these educational settings. All evidence shows that the children perform similarly to or above their peers in other European countries on mathematics, science, and reading literacy. The authors probe further and analyze where there may be differences across the three models in children's performance in these areas and across children with Basque versus Spanish as their first language.

In addition, they report on a study of teenagers' compositions in their three languages, Basque, Spanish, and English. All children were enrolled in D model schools, but came from L1 Basque or L1 Spanish homes. The children's overall achievements in Basque and Spanish were comparable. However, closer analysis of sub-skills in the writing performance showed that on the Basque compositions, while the two groups were comparable on content and organization, the L1 Basque children performed better on vocabulary, use, and mechanics. On the Spanish compositions, the L1 Basque and L1 Spanish children performed in equivalent fashion. On English, the L1 Basque speakers obtained higher scores overall than the L1 Spanish speakers, and the L1 Basque children outperformed the L1 Spanish children on vocabulary, use, and mechanics. The authors discuss their results in terms of the possible relative contributions of language status (majority/minority), relative balance of the languages in the individual bilingual, and 'multilingualism' of the individual; they also comment on the relevance of these data to language assessment and argue for an approach that has a focus on 'multilingualism', involving the whole linguistic repertoire of those being assessed.

(8) A final chapter is concerned with the assessment of bilinguals in educational settings: 'Assessment of Academic Performance: The Impact of No Child Left Behind Policies on Bilingual Education: A ten year retrospective', by Stephen J. Caldas. The issue addressed here is the following:
     Issue 8: Have the treatment and stance towards bilingual children that have been implemented in relation to the No Child Left Behind policies been beneficial or

*detrimental for bilingual children's education? What evidence is there from aca-
demic assessments on the benefits of these policies?*

Caldas provides an authoritative examination of the effects of the
No Child Left Behind legislation in the US on the education of bilingual children. He first provides a history of NCLB legislation, from its
inception, in the Elementary and Secondary Education Act of 1965 to
its emergence as the No Child Left Behind legislation in 2001. He
traces the push and pull of political and philosophical preferences of
the time on education practices affecting children's education, suggesting that while the main focus has been on academic performance,
there has been increasing attention with time on measurable outcomes. Caldas notes that, in principle, NCLB is not necessarily anti-
bilingualism, but there is a strong push to make the attainment of
English in children a priority. He notes that the NCLB has had two
important effects: first, since tests of content areas are administered
in English, they become tests of English proficiency (and, hence, foster
educators' emphasis on learning English), second, educational policy is
being driven by testing policies.

In a revealing study, Caldas examines the performance of bilingual
children (specifically ELL Hispanics) both before and after the NCLB
legislation on national tests of mathematics and reading. He reports that
mathematics scores increased more during the pre-NCLB period (for all
groups, in fact, including non-bilinguals) than since the implementation of NCLB. The increase for Hispanic ELLs was from two and one-
half to seven times *greater* (at grade 4 and grade 8, respectively) during
the period prior to NCLB's implementation than for the period during
which NCLB was the law. For reading, scores for the ELL Hispanics
showed a significant decrease in performance in the eighth-grade scores
during the NCLB period. Furthermore, in fact, there was actually a statistically significant *increase* in the gap between non-ELL and ELL
Hispanic eighth-grade reading scores between 2002 and 2009. So, gaps
between Hispanic ELLs and non-ELLs actually *increased significantly* on
the eighth-grade test.

Such results are a damning indictment of the effects of the NCLB
legislation. When education draws on the resources that a child has
available (e.g. through understanding in the L1), the child is more likely
to succeed academically than when the child is forced to perform in an
L2 for which s/he has a more tenuous grasp.

Issues and Import

These chapters together provide some important directions for movement forward towards more responsive approaches to the assessment

of bilinguals. Among the principles that emerge from this work are the following:

(1)   If at all possible, bilingual children should be tested in both of their languages. When this is not possible, they should be tested in their dominant language.
(2)   When tests do not exist for a particular language, and a researcher wishes to develop a test for that language, it is important to be sensitive to (a) the structure of that language, (b) normal developmental stages children pass through in the acquisition of that language, (c) possible crossover or transfer opportunities between the bilingual's two languages (e.g. the presence of cognates) and (d) possible ramifications for acquisitional patterns associated with growing up in a bilingual community.
(3)   Performance on a test for one language does not necessarily correlate with performance on any other.
(4)   If at all possible, tests should be normed on bilingual children from similar language backgrounds and exposure. If possible, two sets of norms may be appropriate.
(5)   It may be possible to discover means for testing language abilities in bilinguals by testing in the L2. Researchers here have suggested that such testing may take the form of repetition tasks or reaction time measures.
(6)   Even fully fluent end-state bilinguals differ in subtle ways from fluent monolinguals. They may differ in the range and organization of vocabulary and in the processing of language-specific structural features, as in the case of the Spanish object marker *a*.
(7)   The child can build on knowledge of the L1 for the acquisition of L2 abilities, literacy abilities, and academic content. Teachers can make use of the L1 abilities in making bridges to the L2.

One of the resounding themes in these and other works on bilinguals is that difference does not imply deficiency. Yo-Yo Ma plays the cello differently from the way that Jacqueline du Pres did, yet both have been hailed as among the greatest instrumentalists of our time. The manner in which Fred Astaire, Gene Kelly and Mikhail Baryshnikov danced differed dramatically, yet all excelled in their performance. Bilinguals are by definition different from monolinguals; that difference can be celebrated. The chapters in the book argue that we can only do justice to bilingual children and adults if we recognize those differences and draw on them in our treatment and assessment of their abilities.

The chapters in volume 2 attempt to incorporate many of these suggestions into new forms of assessment, to help offer solutions to the many issues raised here.

References

Cummins, J. (1981) *Bilingualism and Minority Language Children*. Ontario: Ontario Institute for Studies in Education.

Dunn, L.M. and Dunn, L.M. (2007) *Peabody Picture Vocabulary Test - III*. Circle Pines, MN: American Guidance Service.

Dunn, L.M., Dunn, L.M., Whetton, C. and Burley, J. (1997) *The British Picture Vocabulary Scale: Second Edition*. NFER-NELSON.

Fenson, L., Marchman, V.A., Thal, D.J., Dale, P.S., Reznick, J.S. and Bates, E. (2007) *MacArthur-Bates Communicative Development Inventories (CDIs), User's Guide and Technical Manual* (2nd edn). Baltimore: Brooks Publishing.

Gathercole, V.C.M. and Thomas, E.M. (2007) *Prawf Geirfa Cymraeg, Fersiwn 7-11*. (Welsh Vocabulary Test, Version 7-11). www.pgc.bangor.ac.uk.

Gathercole, V.C.M. and Thomas, E.M. (2009) Bilingual first-language development: Dominant language takeover, threatened minority language take-up. *Bilingualism: Language and Cognition* 12, 213–237.

Gathercole, V.C.M., Thomas, E.M. and Hughes, E.K. (in press) *Prawf Geirfa Cymraeg, Fersiwn 11–15*. (Welsh Vocabulary Test, Version 11–15).

Grosjean, F. (1982) *Life with Two Languages: An Introduction to Bilingualism*. Cambridge, MA: Harvard University Press.

Guthrie, G. (2003) *1,600 Quotes & Pieces of Wisdom that Just Might Help You Out When You're Stuck in a Moment (and Can't Get Out of It!)*. Lincoln, NE: iUniverse, Inc.

Shah, S. (2011) Brent Paediatric Therapies Department language audit. Report to NHS Brent Community Services.

2 Why Assessment Needs to Take Exposure into Account: Vocabulary and Grammatical Abilities in Bilingual Children

Virginia C. Mueller Gathercole,
Enlli Môn Thomas, Emily J. Roberts,
Catrin O. Hughes and Emma K. Hughes

This chapter argues that bilingual children's level of exposure to each of their languages should be taken into consideration in the norming of language tests. Many normed tests have a single scale against which any child's performance is measured, and that norm is often based on monolingual children learning that language. This chapter examines bilingual children's performance in their two languages on receptive vocabulary and receptive grammar tests and shows that performance is contingent on exposure. For each test, performance relative to exposure to each language and the relation in performance on the two languages was examined. The questions of interest concern how exposure affects timing of development, to what extent performance in the two languages is related, and whether knowledge of a structure in one language can serve to boost performance in the other language. Bilingual Welsh-English-speaking children from 2 years of age to 15 years, from three home language profiles, were tested, as well as monolingual English-speaking children. Data show that exposure is directly related to performance at early ages, although there is some evidence of convergence across participant groups with age. The data also provide little evidence to support direct links between comparable elements in the two languages; any evidence of a correspondence in performance seems to suggest links at some other level, such as at the cognitive or meta-cognitive or meta-linguistic level. Implications for assessment and the design of assessment norms for bilingual children are discussed.

Introduction

It is by now a truism that a bilingual is not two monolinguals in one head. Regardless of the model of language storage, use and acquisition one espouses, there is incontrovertible evidence that at some level and in some ways the fact that bilinguals speak and understand two languages affects their knowledge of language and their processing of language. The languages interact in complex ways, both with each other and with other aspects of cognition. It is not surprising, then, that a bilingual child or adult may not perform in the same way as a monolingual child or adult on any given test assessing language or aspects of cognition drawing on linguistic abilities. The purpose of this chapter is to focus specifically on assessment of linguistic abilities in bilingual children and to examine the ways in which bilingual children's performance may differ from that of monolinguals and how we might alter the way in which we assess bilinguals' abilities to more adequately reflect a true assessment of their abilities. The particular focus here is on early bilinguals – simultaneous bilinguals (or children with two L1s) or early L2-ers (children who begin a second language early in life, e.g. during the preschool years, by 5 years of age or at least during the early school years). We will focus first on how bilingual children's abilities may be different from those of monolingual children, then turn to the purposes of assessment and how the differences between bilinguals and monolinguals may be inadequately addressed in current assessments, and finally turn to some possible solutions to rectify inequities in bilingual assessment. The primary data examined here come from children growing up in the Welsh-English bilingual setting in North Wales.

Bilingual Children's Linguistic Abilities

There are at least four major areas in which we can observe differences in language acquisition and processing in bilingual children in comparison with monolingual children.

(1) First and foremost, and never to be forgotten or downplayed: Bilingual children end up with TWO languages, monolingual children ONE. Regardless of everything else that follows below, this places the bilingual child at a clear long-term advantage over the monolingual child. In the short term, it also means that a child may know something in one language that s/he does not know or knows in a different way in the other language.
(2) Timing of development. Language acquisition depends on hearing input in the given language and interacting with interlocutors speaking that language in real-world contexts that the child interprets in his/her

child-centric way. The child builds a linguistic system based on such input and interaction; the relative frequency of occurrence of such experience influences the timing of acquisition.

(3) Organization of linguistic knowledge. Children's acquisition of language involves building a network of systems for language, including phonological, lexical, syntactic and semantic systems; and at the same time a network of correlated cognitive and social systems. Acquiring two languages makes such systems more complex and richer than when only one language is acquired. The relationship between the bilingual's two languages in this network may influence the nature of the child's knowledge in each language.

(4) Processing of language. Efficient use of language requires ready access to stored knowledge, either when producing or comprehending language. Being ready to use either language at any moment in time means that both languages must be 'on call' in some sense whenever the bilingual is using either language.

All of these are important to keep in mind when considering the proper assessment of bilingual children's abilities in either of their languages. This chapter will focus primarily on point 2, the timing of development, and point 3, the organization of knowledge, and discuss implications for assessment.

Timing of Development

Vocabulary

There is clear evidence in the literature that bilingual children's vocabulary abilities in each of their languages, when measured separately, fall slightly below those of monolingual children in either language (Cobo-Lewis *et al.*, 2002a, 2002b; Cohen, 2006; Gathercole *et al.*, 2008; Gathercole & Thomas, 2009; Hoff *et al.*, 2012; Oller & Pearson, 2002; Pearson & Fernández, 1994; Pearson *et al.*, 1993, 1995; Place & Hoff, 2011; Umbel *et al.*, 1992). (Their total vocabulary scores from their two languages combined add up to or exceed the levels of their monolingual counterparts, however.) This difference appears to be partly attributable to the fact that bilinguals' exposure to their two languages is distributed in nature (Oller, 2005). Language is learned in context, and a bilingual child may hear each language in restricted contexts – in some cases in complementary contexts, in some cases overlapping. For example, a child might hear one language used in the kitchen, another language on a sports field, but at the same time might hear both in a grocery store or in school.

The difference also appears to be due to amount of exposure. If a child hears language A from about half the people s/he hears and language B from the other half, the exposure to each language is half the amount it would have been if s/he heard the same language from all the speakers, as monolinguals do. The effects of exposure on bilinguals' development can be hard to gauge in some cases, since bilingual children often come from distinct socioeconomic or socio-cultural backgrounds from those of their monolingual counterparts. However, in contexts in which monolinguals and bilinguals, and even different types of bilinguals, are comparable in socioeconomic profiles and in socio-cultural background, the effects of exposure can be evaluated more directly. In Wales we have an opportunity to examine exposure fairly directly, as monolinguals and distinct types of bilinguals are growing up in the same socio-cultural context. Within the bilingual population, we are able to divide children according to the language(s) they hear in the home: Some children hear only Welsh at home, some only English, and some both Welsh and English. We now have amassed a considerable amount of data on the vocabulary and grammar abilities of children from a wide range of ages and from these distinct home language backgrounds. The data will show that the differences in exposure to their two languages in the home have clear ramifications for the pace at which children learn the vocabulary and grammar in each of their languages. In this section, the performance on the vocabularies of the two languages is reported.

Method

To gauge vocabulary knowledge of bilingual children in Wales, we administered receptive vocabulary tests in English and Welsh to children between the ages of 2 and 15. For English, the BPVS (British Picture Vocabulary Scales, Dunn, et al., 1997) was used, and for Welsh, the original 240 words gathered for the development of the *Prawf Geirfa Cymraeg* (Gathercole & Thomas, 2007; Gathercole et al., 2008) were tested. The original 240 words were chosen from eight frequency levels (Ellis et al., 2001) with the constraint that they were not borrowings (or cognates) from English (see Gathercole & Thomas, 2007, for more detail). Bilingual children were administered both tests, monolingual English speakers were administered the BPVS only. (Monolingual Welsh speakers are rare, possibly non-existent.)

Participants

For the BPVS, 427 children were tested, including monolinguals ($N = 96$) and bilinguals ($N = 331$), and for the PGC, all 331 of the bilinguals were tested. The children came from four distinct home language groups, according to the language(s) reported by parents to be the language(s) spoken by them to their children in the home: monolingual English ('Mon E'), bilinguals with only English at home ('OEH'), bilinguals with both Welsh and English at home ('WEH') and bilinguals with only Welsh at home ('OWH').

Children came from four distinct age groups, 2–3 (mean age 3;2, range 2;0–4;0), 4–5 (mean age 4;11, range 4;1–6;7), 7–8 (mean age 8;0, range 7;0–8;11) and 13–15 (mean age 14;7, range 13;0–15;8). The number of children tested at each age is shown in Table 2.1 by home language. The breakdown of ages, with means and median ages for each home language group at each age, is shown in Table 2.2.

Procedure

The tests were administered in conjunction with a battery of other tests exploring general cognitive abilities and performance on executive function tasks, not reported here (see Gathercole *et al.*, 2010; Gathercole *et al.*, in submission). Tests were administered on two or three different days, the English and Welsh language tests always on distinct days. The order of testing for English and Welsh language tests was counter-balanced across participants.

Table 2.1 Participants, English and Welsh vocabulary measures, by age group and home language

Age	MON E	OEH	WEH	OWH	TOT
2–3	31	24	22	33	110
4–5	20	27	26	23	96
7–8	25	29	25	33	112
13–15	20	25	30	34	109
	96	103	103	125	427

MON E = monolingual English (only tested in English); OEH = bilingual with only English at home; WEH = bilingual with Welsh and English at home; OWH = bilingual with only Welsh at home

Table 2.2 Mean (and median) ages for participants, English and Welsh vocabulary measures, by age group and home language

Age	MON E	OEH	WEH	OWH	TOT
2–3	3;5	3;0	3;1	3;2	3;2
	(3;6)	(3;1)	(3;1)	(3;2)	(3;3)
4–5	4;9	4;11	5;0	4;10	4;11
	(4;7)	(4;11)	(5;1)	(4;9)	(4;10)
7–8	7;9	8;2	8;1	8;1	8;0
	(7;7)	(8;3)	(8;2)	(8;1)	(8;1)
13–15	14;7	14;7	14;6	14;9	14;7
	(14;10)	(15;0)	(14;7)	(14;9)	(14;9)

MON E = monolingual English; OEH = bilingual with only English at home; WEH = bilingual with Welsh and English at home; OWH = bilingual with only Welsh at home

Results
English, BPVS

An ANOVA in which age group and home language were entered as variables revealed that performance on the BPVS differed significantly by age, F (3, 426) = 1237.6, $p < 0.001$, and by home language, F (3, 411) = 30.2, $p < 0.001$. All age groups performed significantly differently, all pairwise comparisons $p < 0.001$, all Scheffe's multiple comparisons $p < 0.001$. All home languages differed significantly when submitted to pairwise comparisons (all ps < 0.001 except for Mon E vs OEH, which differed at $p = 0.011$, and OEH vs WEH, which differed at $p = 0.007$). Under Scheffe's multiple comparisons, only OWH differed significantly from all other home language groups, all ps < 0.001.

Performance by age and home language is shown in Figure 2.1. There was no significant interaction of Age X Home Language, but the results in Figure 2.1 show a trend towards possible convergence across home languages with age. To explore this possibility further, separate ANOVAs were computed at each age for the effects of home language. The results are shown in Table 2.3. Comparisons across the ages show that, whereas at the youngest age, home language groups tend to perform differently, as children get older, the home language groups gradually become less distinguishable. Thus, at age 2–3, all home language groups are distinguishable except for the OEH and WEH groups. By ages 4–5 and 7–8, OEH children are no longer significantly different from Mon E children, and WEH tend to perform only marginally differently from the Mon E and OEH children. By ages 13–15, the only group that shows any significantly different performance from the others is the OWH group,

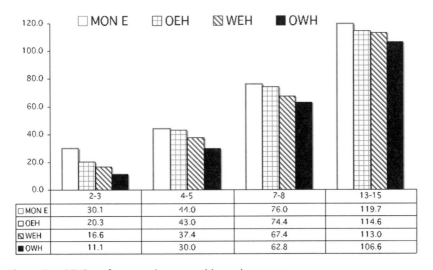

Figure 2.1 BPVS performance by age and home language

Table 2.3 ANOVA by age group for home language effects, BPVS

	ANOVA			Pairwise comparisons		Scheffé's multiple comparisons	
	F	df	p		p		p
2–3	29.29	3,106	0.000	Mon E > OEH , WEH , OWH	0.000	Mon E > OEH , WEH , OWH	0.001
				OEH > WEH , OWH	0.000	Mon E > WEH , OWH	0.000
				WEH > OWH	0.016	OEH > OWH	0.001
4–5	7.29	3,9	0.000	Mon E , OEH > WEH , OWH	0.000	Mon E , OEH > WEH , OWH	0.002
				WEH > OWH	0.026		
				Mon E ? WEH	0.057		
				OEH ? WEH	0.080		
7–8	6.08	3,108	0.001	Mon E > WEH	0.027	Mon E > OWH	0.005
				Mon E > OEH , WEH , OWH	0.000	OEH > OWH	0.012
				OEH > OWH	0.001		
				OEH ? WEH	0.061		
13–15	4.20	3,105	0.008	Mon E > OEH , WEH , OWH	0.001	Mon E > OWH	0.011
				OEH > WEH	0.028		
				Mon E ? WEH	0.089		
				WEH ? OWH	0.065		

which, under the more stringent Scheffe test, only differ at this age from the Mon E children. Thus, early differences across groups get neutralized with age.

Welsh, PGC

An ANOVA in which age group and home language were entered as variables revealed that performance on the PGC differed significantly by age, F (3, 319) = 784.4, $p < 0.001$, and by home language, F (2, 319) = 44.4, $p < 0.001$. All age groups performed significantly differently, all pairwise comparisons $p < 0.001$, all Scheffe's multiple comparisons $p < 0.001$. All home languages differed significantly when submitted to pairwise comparisons, all ps < 0.001. Under Scheffe's multiple comparisons, all home language groups differed significantly (all ps < 0.001, except for WEH and OWH, which differed at $p = 0.031$).

There was also a significant interaction of Home Language X Age, F (6, 319) = 5.0, $p < 0.001$. Performance by age and home language is shown in Figure 2.2. Follow-up ANOVAs were computed at each age. The results are shown in Table 2.4. As in the case of the English vocabulary performance, performance on Welsh shows changes with age in the comparability of home language groups. At the youngest age, age 2–3, the OWH children significantly outperform both the OEH and WEH groups, whose performance is indistinguishable. By age 4–5, the WEH children outperfom the OEH children; by the more stringent Scheffe's test of multiple comparisons, the WEH children are only marginally different from the OWH children by this age. By age 7–8, the WEH children's performance matches that of the OWH children, with the OEH children clearly distinct still from both of these groups. By ages 13–15, the OEH children are closing the gap with the WEH children; they are significantly different from the OWH children, but, by Scheffe's

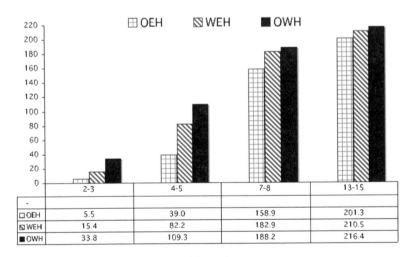

	2-3	4-5	7-8	13-15
▢ OEH	5.5	39.0	158.9	201.3
◩ WEH	15.4	82.2	182.9	210.5
■ OWH	33.8	109.3	188.2	216.4

Figure 2.2 PGC performance by age and home language

Table 2.4 ANOVA by age group for home language effects, PGC

	ANOVA			Pairwise comparisons		Scheffe's multiple comparisons	
	F	df	p		p		p
2–3	39.28	2,76	0.000	WEH < OWH	0.011	WEH < OWH	0.037
				OEH < OWH	0.000	OEH < OWH	0.000
4–5	18.15	2,73	0.000	WEH < OWH	0.026	OEH < OWH	0.000
				OEH < WEH , OWH	0.000	OEH < WEH	0.002
						WEH ~ OWH	0.083
7–8	10.84	2,84	0.000	OEH < OWH	0.000	OEH < OWH	0.000
				OEH < WEH	0.001	OEH < WEH	0.004
13–15	5.72	2,86	0.005	OEH < OWH	0.001	OEH < OWH	0.005
				OEH < WEH	0.048		

comparisons, they are no longer distinct from the WEH children. Thus, as is true for English, early differences across groups in performance on Welsh vocabulary tend to neutralize with age. (See qualification below regarding OEH children from communities with lower levels of Welsh speakers.)

These data together show consistent differences in vocabulary performance according to language exposure. Those children with more exposure to English advance earlier than those with less exposure; those children with more exposure to Welsh advance earlier than those with less exposure. Over time, as all groups gain more experience with both languages, there is a tendency across groups to become less distinguishable, i.e. more similar in performance.

Grammatical abilities

In order to similarly examine children's knowledge of grammatical structures in each language, we developed receptive grammatical tests in each language that covered roughly comparable structures in the two languages. They were 'roughly comparable' in the sense that the structures expressed comparable functions, not necessarily in the formation of the structure itself (see Gathercole, 2009a, for elaboration).

Method
Stimuli

Thirteen sets of structures were chosen for inclusion in the tests, namely the following:

• Active sentences
• Negation

- Passive (truncated)
- Comparative
- Superlative
- Present perfect
- Future
- Time conjunctions (*before/after/until*)
- Relative clause, OS
- Relative clause, SS
- Relative clause, SO
- Quantification, universal or exhaustive (*every, both*)
- Quantification, existential or non-exhaustive (*some, not all*)

An example of each type of structure for English and Welsh is shown in Table 2.5.

Table 2.5 Types of structures tested in receptive grammar tasks

Structure type	English Examples	Welsh examples
Active	The elephant smelled the horse.	Gwnaeth yr eliffant ogleuo'r ceffyl.
Negation	The goats aren't eating.	Tydi'r geifr ddim yn bwyta.
Passive (Truncated)	The clown was pushed.	Cafodd y clown ei wthio.
Comparative	The tree is taller than the house.	Mae'r goeden yn dalach na'r ty.
Superlative	The apple is lowest.	Yr afal sydd isaf.
Present perfect	He has jumped.	Mae o wedi neidio.
Future	The ducks will jump over the rock.	Mi wneith y hwyaid neidio dros y garreg.
Time conjunction (*before/after/until*)	Before the teacher fell, she took her hat off.	Cyn i'r athrawes ddisgyn, mi dynnodd hi ei het.
Relative clause, OS	A circle covers the box that has a ring in it.	Mae're cylch yn gorchuddio'r bocs sydd efo modrwy ynddo.
Relative clause, SS	The donkey that kicked a cow was wearing socks.	Roedd yr asyn naeth gicio'r fuwch yn gwisgo sanau.
Relative clause, SO	The donkey that a cow held had a purple tail.	Roedd yr asyn yr oedd buwch yn ei afael efo cynffon biws.
Quantifier, universal / exhaustive (*every, both*)	Every princess is on a tractor.	Mae pob tywysoges ar dractor.
Quantifier, existential / non- exhaustive (*not all, some*)	Some of the dancers are wearing dresses.	Mae rhai o'r dawnswyr yn gwisgo ffrogiau.

Two versions of the tests, A and B, were prepared for both languages, so that a given child would not receive the same pictures or translation-equivalent sentences across the two languages. In each version, each type of grammatical structure was tested with three trials in a forced-choice picture task, with four picture choices for each trial. The lexical items appearing in versions A and B were the same, but their occurrence was balanced so that they would be heard on distinct trials and in distinct structures across the versions. Approximately half the children received version A in English and B in Welsh, and half version B in English and A in Welsh.

Procedure

For each trial, a set of four computerized pictures was presented, and the child was asked to pick the picture that went best with the sentence s/he heard. All verbal stimuli were presented aurally. Five practice trials unrelated to the structures of interest were administered initially, in the relevant language, to familiarize the child with the procedure.

Participants

For the English receptive grammar task, 376 children were tested, including monolinguals and bilinguals, and for the Welsh receptive grammar task, all 278 of the bilinguals were tested. The children came from four distinct home language groups, according to the language(s) reported by parents to be the language(s) spoken by them to children in the home: monolingual English, bilinguals with only English at home ('OEH'), bilinguals with both Welsh and English at home ('WEH'), and bilinguals with only Welsh at home ('OWH').

Children came from four distinct age groups, 2–3 (mean age 3;3, range 2;1–4;0), 4–5 (mean age 5;0, range 4;1–6;8), 7–8 (mean age 8;1, range 7;0–8;11) and 13–15 (mean age 14;8, range 13;0–15;8). The number of children tested at each age is shown in Table 2.6 by home language. The breakdown of ages, with means and median ages for each home language group at each age, is shown in Table 2.7.

Results

English receptive grammar

An ANOVA in which age group and home language were entered as variables revealed that performance on the English receptive grammar test differed significantly by age, $F (3, 360) = 489.5$, $p < 0.001$, and by home language, $F (3, 360) = 14.73$, $p < 0.001$. All age groups performed significantly differently, all pairwise comparisons $p < 0.001$, all Scheffe's multiple comparisons $p < 0.001$. The Mon E speakers performed significantly differently from all bilingual groups, and the OEH speakers outperformed the OWH speakers: pairwise comparisons: Mon E vs OEH $p = 0.002$, Mon E vs WEH $p < 0.001$, Mon E vs OWH $p < 0.001$, OEH vs OWH $p = 0.007$. (Under Scheffe's multiple

Table 2.6 Participants, English and Welsh receptive grammar measures, by age group and home language

Age	MON E	OEH	WEH	OWH	TOT
2–3	23	11	18	22	74
4–5	38	25	20	23	106
7–8	17	30	22	33	102
13–15	20	18	25	31	94
	98	84	85	109	376

MON E = monolingual English (only tested in English); OEH = bilingual with only English at home; WEH = bilingual with Welsh and English at home; OWH = bilingual with only Welsh at home

Table 2.7 Mean (and median) ages for participants, English and Welsh receptive grammar measures, by age group and home language

Age	MON E	OEH	WEH	OWH	TOT
2–3	3;6	3;2	3;1	3;1	3;3
	(3;7)	(3;2)	(3;0)	(3;1)	(3;3)
4–5	5;0	5;0	5;1	4;10	5;0
	(4;10)	(5;0)	(5;3)	(4;9)	(4;11)
7–8	7;9	8;1	8;1	8;2	8;1
	(7;7)	(8;2)	(8;1)	(8;2)	(8;1)
13–15	14;7	14;7	14;8	14;9	14;8
	(14;10)	(15;1)	(14;11)	(14;9)	(14;10)

MON E = monolingual English; OEH = bilingual with only English at home; WEH = bilingual with Welsh and English at home; OWH = bilingual with only Welsh at home

comparisons, there was a near–significant difference between the OEH and OWH groups, $p = 0.073$.)

There was also a significant interaction of Home Language X Age, $F(9,360) = 2.15$, $p = 0.025$. Performance by age and home language is shown in Figure 2.3. For follow-up analyses, separate ANOVAs were computed at each age for the effects of home language. The results are shown in Table 2.8. Comparisons across the ages show that, whereas at the youngest age, home language groups tended to perform differently, as children got older, the home language groups gradually became less distinguishable. Thus, at ages 2–3 and 4–5, Mon E children generally performed significantly differently from OEH, WEH and OWH children (or, by the more stringent Scheffe's Multiple Comparisons, from WEH and OWH children). By age 7–8, OEH children no longer performed differently from Mon E children, but WEH and OWH children (or the OWH children only, by Scheffe's Multiple Comparisons) still performed less well than the Mon E children. By ages

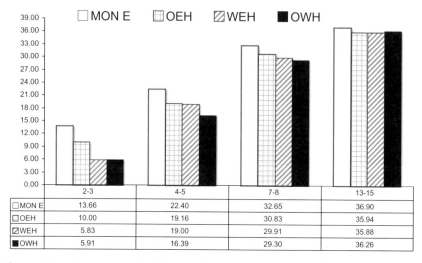

	MON E	OEH	WEH	OWH
	2-3	4-5	7-8	13-15
☐ MON E	13.66	22.40	32.65	36.90
☐ OEH	10.00	19.16	30.83	35.94
☑ WEH	5.83	19.00	29.91	35.88
■ OWH	5.91	16.39	29.30	36.26

Figure 2.3 Performance on English receptive grammar by age and home language

Table 2.8 ANOVA by Age Group for home language effects, English receptive grammar

	ANOVA			Pairwise comparisons					Scheffe's multiple comparisons		
	F	df	p					p			p
2–3	7.56	3,70	0.000	Mon E	>		WEH ,	OWH 0.000	Mon E > WEH		0.003
									Mon E >	OWH	0.002
4–5	5.12	3,102	0.002	Mon E	> OEH			0.037	Mon E >	OWH	0.003
				Mon E	>	WEH		0.042			
				Mon E	>		OWH	0.000			
7–8	2.66	3,98	0.052	Mon E	>	WEH		0.043	Mon E >	OWH	0.068
				Mon E	>		OWH	0.008			
13–15	0.65	3,90	n.s.								

13–15, all children performed in an equivalent fashion. Thus, early differences across groups became neutralized with age.

Welsh receptive grammar

Performance by age and home language is shown for Welsh in Figure 2.4. An ANOVA in which age group and home language were entered as variables revealed that performance on the Welsh receptive grammar test differed significantly by age, $F (3, 266) = 325.2, p < 0.001$, and by home language, $F (2,266) = 8.98, p < 0.001$. All age groups performed significantly differently, all pairwise comparisons $p < 0.001$, all Scheffe's multiple comparisons $p < 0.001$. The OWH speakers performed significantly differently

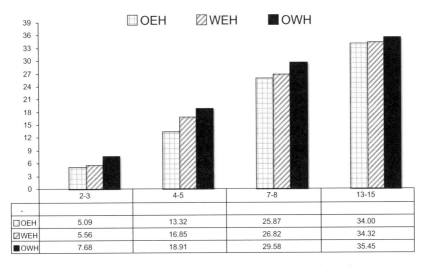

	2-3	4-5	7-8	13-15
☐OEH	5.09	13.32	25.87	34.00
▨WEH	5.56	16.85	26.82	34.32
■OWH	7.68	18.91	29.58	35.45

Figure 2.4 Performance on Welsh receptive grammar by age and home language

from the other bilingual groups: OWH vs. WEH $p = 0.010$, OWH vs OEH $p < 0.001$. (Under Scheffe's multiple comparisons, OWH outperformed both WEH and OEH children, $p = 0.009$ and $p < 0.001$, respectively).

Although there was not a significant interaction of Home Language X Age, to explore the results by age group, separate ANOVAs were computed at each age to examine effects of home language in more detail. The results are shown in Table 2.9. Comparisons across the ages show that, first, at the youngest age, there was no observable difference across groups. This is likely attributable to the fact that scores at this age were near the floor. At ages 4–5 and 7–8 the differences across home language groups were most apparent, with OEH children most clearly distinct from OWH children, with the WEH children performing between these two. By ages 13–15, differences across groups were no longer significant. Thus, again, early differences across groups appeared to get neutralized with age.

Table 2.9 ANOVA by age group for home language effects, Welsh receptive grammar

	ANOVA			*Pairwise comparisons*				*Scheffe's multiple comparisons*			
	F	df	p				p				p
2–3	0.76	2,48	n.s.								
4–5	7.65	2,65	0.001	OEH		< OWH	0.000	OEH		< OWH	.001
				OEH	< WEH		0.022	OEH	~ WEH		.071
7–8	3.93	2,82	0.024	OEH		< OWH	0.008	OEH		< OWH	.030
				WEH	~ OWH		0.069				
13–15	0.83	2,71	n.s.								

These data regarding children's receptive grammatical abilities reveal, like the data on vocabulary knowledge, that the pace of development is directly tied to the amount of exposure the child has to each language: Those with the greatest exposure to English perform better earlier than those with less exposure; those with the greatest exposure to Welsh perform better earlier than those with less exposure. Children's abilities across home language groups appear to become more similar with age, as children gain the knowledge of the given structures. It is worth noting that the abilities across home language groups appear to become more similar at an earlier age for grammatical knowledge than is the case with vocabulary abilities. There are at least two possible reasons for this. First, the nature of the child's exposure to vocabulary and grammatical structures is different. Acquiring vocabulary and acquiring grammatical structures involve distinct type-token ratios: vocabulary acquisition generally involves exposure to many types [many different words], and few tokens for each type, whereas grammar acquisition generally involves exposure to relatively few types [few different structures], and many tokens for each type. In the acquisition of grammatical structures the child appears to abstract or consolidate a structure once s/he has gained a critical mass of experience. The multiple token exposure that grammatical forms afford may help ensure accumulation of that critical mass, so with time, the knowledge across home language groups becomes quite comparable.

A second possible reason why home language differences become less distinguishable in relation to these grammatical structures than in relation to vocabulary may have to do with the fact that the tests used here were receptive. There may be a more complex set of factors that contribute to understanding sentences than understanding words: grammatical understanding involves not only the structure involved, but also any cognitive, pragmatic and lexical knowledge that contributes to the semantic import of a sentence. One must draw on all of these to interpret a sentence. As children's cognitive, pragmatic and lexical knowledge are developing in tandem with their grammatical development, it is possible that this also furthers greater comparability across home language groups earlier in a receptive grammar task than in a receptive lexical task. (See further discussion below.) It is quite possible that in a productive grammar task less convergence across home language groups might be observed.

Organization of Knowledge in Bilinguals

There is considerable evidence that simultaneous and early bilinguals' linguistic systems, particularly the morpho-syntactic systems, develop separately from very early (Meisel, 1989, 2001; Döpke, 1998, 2000; Paradis & Genesee, 1996; Hulk & Müller, 2000). At the same time, there is ample evidence as well that the two systems must eventually be linked, as crosslinguistic priming studies show that forms from one language call up related forms in the speaker's other language (Dijkstra & Van Heuven, 1998; Grosjean, 1998, 2001; Dijkstra & van Hell, 2003). This raises the question about the extent to which a bilingual child's performance in one language can inform us about either the child's general linguistic abilities or his/her abilities in the other language. To examine this issue, let us look again at the Welsh-English children's vocabulary and grammatical abilities. By comparing each child's performance across the two languages, we can gain some insights.

Vocabulary in two languages

First, the above children's vocabulary scores in their two languages were compared. Children's performance on the BPVS and the PGC is plotted by age in Figures 2.5 to 2.8. On these scatter plots BPVS scores appear on the X axis and PGC scores on the Y axis. (In order to include the Mon E children on these plots for comparison, the Mon E children were entered by assigning them, arbitrarily, a score of –10 on the PGC, to distinguish them from the

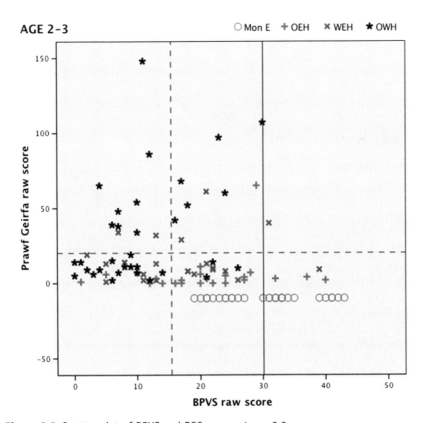

Figure 2.5 Scatter plot of BPVS and PGC scores at age 2-3

AGE 4-5

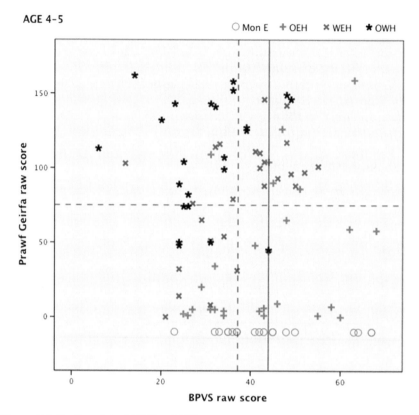

Figure 2.6 Scatter plot of BPVS and PGC scores at age 4-5

children who were actually administered that test.) On the plots, the vertical solid line indicates the mean score for Mon E participants on the BPVS, and the dotted lines, vertical and horizontal, indicate the location of the bilinguals' mean scores for each test at the given age.

Correlational analyses of scores on the English vocabulary test, the BPVS, and the Welsh vocabulary test, the PGC, were computed for each age group. The scores at ages 2–3, 4–5 and 7–8 were not significantly correlated. This suggests that vocabulary abilities in the two languages are not related at these ages. At ages 13–15, the scores did correlate significantly, Pearson's $r = 0.229, p = 0.031$.

The scatter plots provide a visual confirmation of these results and of a number of facts: First, the scatter plots clearly demonstrate that at the younger ages, children can perform well in one language while at the same time performing poorly in their other language. Some bilingual children can be described either as dominant in Welsh or as dominant in English. For example, the bilingual children coming from OWH homes tend to fall, at least at the younger ages, towards the top left quadrant of each plot, indicating rela-

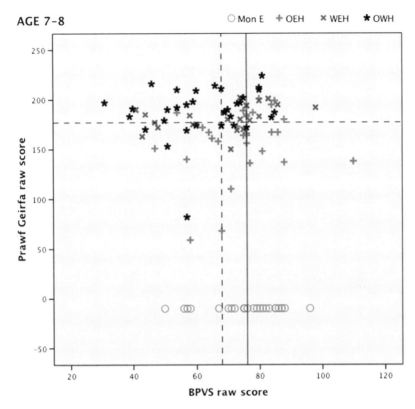

Figure 2.7 Scatter plot of BPVS and PGC scores at age 7-8

tively higher scores on Welsh and lower scores on English; bilingual children coming from OEH homes, in contrast, tend to fall towards the lower right quadrant, indicating relatively higher scores in English and lower scores in Welsh. At the same time, those bilingual children coming from WEH homes can be seen to more generally fall in a more central area of the graphs, indicating more balanced abilities in their two languages. This difference in distribution and abilities is highly relevant to assessment of bilingual children, to which we return below. The scatter plots also demonstrate clearly in the case of English that the Mon E children start out in advance of their bilingual peers at age 2–3, but that with increasing age the bilinguals gradually fall within a similar range of scores as the monolinguals.

On vocabulary, then, at least at preschool and primary school ages, performance on one language can tell us nothing about the child's performance on the other language. By the teen years, there is a significant correlation in the child's performance on the two languages. This correlation could mean that the vocabularies in the two languages by these ages are linked; however, alternatively, it may be reflective of general vocabulary-learning abilities (if

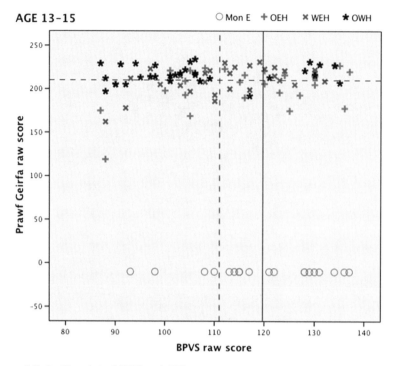

Figure 2.8 Scatter plot of BPVS and PGC scores at age 13-15

a child is a good word learner in one language, s/he is a good word learner in the other), rather than necessarily implicating direct links between the vocabularies of the two languages.

Grammatical knowledge in the two languages

Children's grammatical abilities in their two languages were similarly compared. Scatter plots at each age are shown in Figures 2.9 to 2.12. (Again, in order to include the Mon E children on these plots for comparison, they were entered by assigning them, arbitrarily, a score of –2 on the Welsh grammatical test.)

Correlational analyses of scores on the two tests were computed for each age group. (Children whose scores were zero on both grammar tasks ($N = 13$ of the 2- to 3-year-olds) were eliminated from these analyses.) There were significant correlations between the total scores on the two tests at ages 2–3, $r = 0.552$, $p = 0.000$, at 7–8, $r = 0.353$, $p = 0.001$ and at 13–15, $r = 0.384$, $p = 0.001$, but not at age 4–5, $r = 0.144$, n.s.

In order to understand these overall correlations, possible correlations at each age on the sub-tasks were examined. It could be that children were 'bootstrapping' from one language to the other, especially in cases in which English and Welsh were comparable in structure. If so, the prediction would

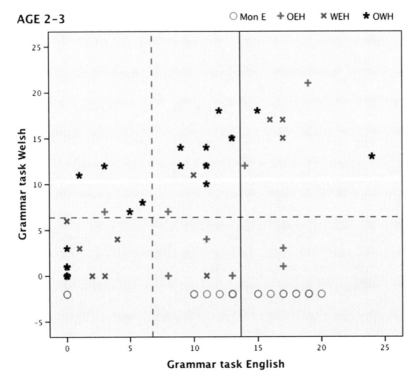

Figure 2.9 Scatter plot of English and Welsh grammar scores at age 2-3

be that there would be significant correlations on structures that were similar across the two languages, but not on structures that were dissimilar. If, on the other hand, correlations occurred in cases in which the structures were dissimilar, this would suggest that some other factor – e.g. requisite cognitive preparation for use of the structure in question or a more general linguistic advancement, such as expanded MLU length – might account for correlations in performance.

There were significant correlations on the following sub-scores:

- At age 2–3: comparatives $r = 0.405$, $p = 0.012$; time conjunctions $r = 0.481$, $p = 0.002$; SO relatives: $r = 0.480$, $p = 0.002$; future $r = 0.395$, $p = 0.014$.
- At age 4–5: passive $r = 0.241$, $p = 0.050$; comparatives $r = 0.279$, $p = 0.022$; existential/non-exhaustive quantification $r = 0.319$, $p = 0.010$; OS relatives $r = 0.276$, $p = 0.024$.
- At age 7–8: actives: $r = 0.296$, $p = 0.006$; existential/non-exhaustive quantification $r = 0.441$, $p = 0.0-00$; SO relatives $r = 0.241$, $p = 0.029$.
- At age 13–15: passive $r = 0.297$, $p = 0.010$; present perfect $r = 0.299$, $p = 0.010$; universal/exhaustive quantification $r = 0.410$, $p = 0.000$.

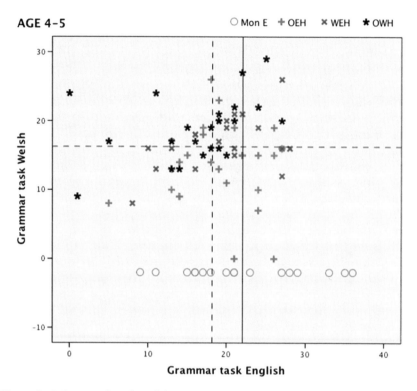

Figure 2.10 Scatter plot of English and Welsh grammar scores at age 4-5

Interestingly and importantly, for some of these constructions, English and Welsh structures are similar in linguistic formation, and for others they are drastically different. The following appear quite comparable in form: The comparative in both languages involves the use of a suffix on the adjective (-*er* in English, -*ach* in Welsh) followed by a standard marker (*than* in English, *na* in Welsh) introducing the standard of comparison; quantifiers in both languages are pre-nominal (*every N, pob N; some of the N, rhai o'r N*).

In contrast, the following are quite distinct: The passive in English is formed with an auxiliary *be* or *get* followed by the past participle of the main verb, whereas the passive in Welsh is formed with the auxiliary *cael* 'get' followed by the verb modified by a possessive adjective – the Welsh passive in Table 2.5 is literally 'got the clown his push'. Relatives are also constructed differently. For SO relatives, in English the subject is followed by the relative clause introduced by the (optional) complementizer *that,* and there is no resumptive pronoun for the direct object in the embedded clause, as in (1):

(1)   a. The donkey [that a cow held _____] had a purple tail.
      b. The card [that a painting showed _____] had a flower on it.

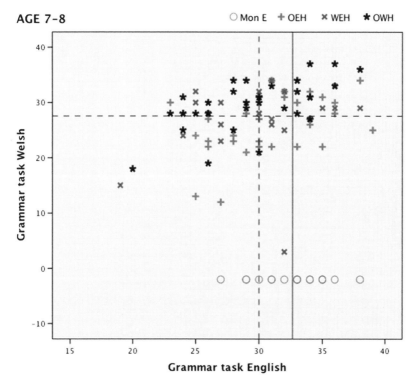

Figure 2.11 Scatter plot of English and Welsh grammar scores at age 7-8

In the equivalent sentences in Welsh, as in (2), there may or may not be a complementizer (here *yr*) and there may be a resumptive pronoun in the form of a possessive adjective (*ei*) modifying the embedded verb, as in (2):

(2) a. Roedd yr asyn   [yr   oedd buwch yn ei   afael]   efo cynffon biws.
       was   the donkey [COMP was cow   PRT him   hold]   with tail   purple

   b. Roedd y cerdyn [roedd y   llun   yn ei   ddangos] efo blodyn arno.
       was   the card   [was   the picture PRT it   show]   with flower on

Similarly, with OS relatives, English uses a complementizer, as in (3), whereas Welsh may not, as in (4):

(3) A pig smelled the elephant [that _____ was eating an orange].
(4) Naeth y   mochyn ogleuo'r llyffant [____ oedd yn   bwyta oren   ].
      did   the pig   smell-the elephant [____ was   PRT eat   orange]

   Another case of a difference is in the formation of the present perfect. English uses a form of the auxiliary *have* in combination with the past

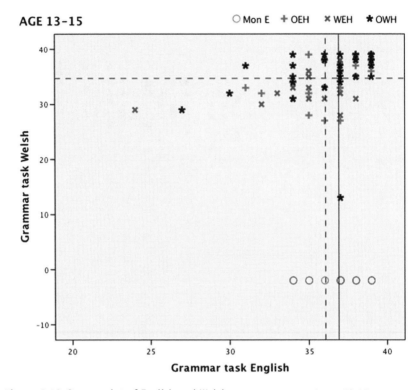

Figure 2.12 Scatter plot of English and Welsh grammar scores at age 13-15

participle of the verb (e.g. *eaten*), whereas Welsh uses the auxiliary *bod* 'be' in combination with the preposition *wedi* 'after' and the infinitival form of the verb.

Finally, in some cases in which correlations occurred, there appears to be both some similarity and some difference in the English and Welsh structures. For example, for structures involving time conjunctions, English and Welsh both have introductory conjunctions (*before, cyn*), but English *before* usually introduces a finite clause (*before the teacher fell...*), while Welsh *cyn* introduces a non-finite structure (*cyn i'r athrawes ddisgyn....* 'before to the teacher falling....' [cf. *prior to the teacher falling....*]).

Thus, the correlations that hold at the different ages on substructures of the two languages do so for both comparable structures (e.g. the comparative) and dissimilar structures (e.g. relative clauses, passives). (See Gathercole *et al.*, in press, for further elaboration.) This suggests that, rather than children bootstrapping from the syntactic structures of one language to the other, there may be a certain cognitive preparedness or a general linguistic preparedness that allows children to map some cognitive understanding or linguistic advance they have gained with the linguistic means for expressing that in each language. For example, for proper use of the comparative (in any language), one must come to a certain level of appreciation of comparison between entities, and of the relative position of two values on a given scale (see Gathercole, 2009b). For the proper use of relative clauses, there must be among other things an ability to hold multiple components of a sentence in memory and an ability to coordinate multiple grammatical/theta roles for nominal elements expressed in the sentence or a meta-linguistic appreciation that such multiple relations can hold within a single sentence. That such advances should affect advances in both languages would not be surprising.

These results concerning the relative grammatical abilities in the two languages reveal two major findings. First, the correlations show a somewhat greater relationship between children's grammatical abilities in the two languages than we observed for their two vocabularies. Correlations on total scores held at all ages except for 4–5; and correlations between some substructures were found at every age. This may suggest a closer link between grammatical abilities in the child's two languages than between his/her two vocabularies.

However, secondly, the correlational data also suggest that the relationship may occur via some route other than through some direct linkage between the morpho-syntactic structures of the two languages. The underlying cognitive or linguistic preparation needed for the acquisition of the structure in question is likely to contribute to developments in both languages. Thus, for example, it may not be that a child does well on the comparative in English BECAUSE s/he knows the comparative in Welsh; rather, s/he may do well on the comparative in both languages because of some other cognitive or linguistic achievement that underlies its use in both languages. It should be noted that the design of the grammar tests intentionally focused on functionally comparable structures in the two languages. It did not include structures that were unique to one of the two languages (e.g. grammatical gender in Welsh *et al.*, 2007). It is possible that if such more language-specific structures were included, we would observe lower correlations in overall performance on the two languages.

Purposes of Assessment and Appropriateness for Bilinguals

Data such as those presented above have important implications for the assessment of children who are growing up as bilinguals. The implications apply both to testing for children's linguistic abilities and to testing for a myriad of other reasons. In the section that follows, the uses of assessment measures are explored, and some suggestions are made for accommodations needed to allow for the nature of bilingual development.

Uses of assessment

There are vast numbers of purposes for which professionals use standardized (and non-standardized) tests, whether of children's vocabulary or grammatical abilities or of abilities beyond these – cognitive attainment, academic abilities, literacy abilities and the like. We can group these uses into purposes related to the assessment of linguistic abilities and purposes that draw on linguistic abilities for performance in another realm. Let us start with the latter.

Non-language-related purposes of assessment

Tests that aim at providing information on a child's conceptual knowledge or academic abilities, first of all, must be administered through the medium of language. Academic abilities, e.g. in mathematics, history, science and the like, are also usually probed through language. It goes without saying that if a child does not understand the language of the instructions or the language of a question, s/he cannot demonstrate knowledge in the area. To gain a true measure of a child's abilities in any of such academic areas, assessment should ideally occur in the language in which the child is most proficient.

Testing conceptual knowledge is a little more tricky. There are some tests that attempt to bypass the effect of linguistic knowledge on cognitive performance – e.g. Raven's Progressive Matrices (Raven *et al.*, 2004). But when particular concepts are the focus of the test, the probing of those concepts often occurs through language. This is because a child's linguistic knowledge, especially vocabulary knowledge, is closely tied with the child's conceptual knowledge: If a child knows the word for a type of object or action or state, one can surmise that s/he also has (non-linguistic) knowledge of that category of objects or actions or states; if a child knows different words for different types of objects or actions, then one can infer that s/he understands differences across types of objects or actions and so forth. Vocabulary measures are often used to gain a 'window' into that conceptual knowledge (or are often included within measures of 'cognitive' knowledge, as in the McCarthy, 1972, and the Reynell, 1987).

When dealing with monolingual children, such a leap from measurement of vocabulary abilities to inferences about cognitive abilities is fairly warranted. When dealing with bilingual children, on the other hand, such a leap should be taken with extreme caution and is generally invalid if based on only one of the child's languages. First, as demonstrated above, knowing a bilingual child's vocabulary abilities in only one of his/her languages will provide a skewed picture of that child's abilities (Oller & Pearson, 2002), since a child may know the words for some concepts only in the other language.

Furthermore, the manner in which the bilingual's two languages 'carve up' the conceptual space may be drastically different (Bowerman, 1996a, 1996b; Bowerman & Choi, 2001; Elston-Gathercole *et al.*, 2011; Gathercole & Moawad, 2010; Güttler & Williams, 2008; Malt *et al.*, 2003; Pavlenko, 2009). What may be a single concept in one language (e.g. *wall* in English) may be cut into finer distinctions in another language (Spanish distinguishes *pared* 'wall' inside a building, *muro* 'wall' outside, as a stone wall, *muralla* 'wall' as around a city); Spanish *dedo* encompasses both fingers and toes, while English separates *fingers* from *toes*; and so forth. Thus, if a Spanish-background child picks a picture of toes when asked to find the 'fingers', or a Welsh-background child chooses a picture of boots when asked to find the 'shoes', it is likely that this is because their other language groups fingers and toes or shoes and boots together. It does not necessarily imply anything about that child's knowledge on a non-linguistic level about fingers and toes or about shoes and boots (see Gathercole, 2010; Gathercole & Moawad, 2010).

These differences in how the conceptual space is carved up by the language go well beyond the vocabulary as well. Compare English *a X/one X* with Spanish *un X*. In English *a X* encodes non-specific reference, while *one X* is a quantifier phrase indicating number. If I tell you that I am going shopping for 'a red dress', and then you find out that I actually ended up coming home with two red dresses, you would probably not feel I had deceived you. In contrast, if I tell you that I am going shopping for 'one red dress', you may well feel as if I had deceived you if you found out I actually ended up with two. Contrast this with what it is possible to encode in Spanish. In Spanish, the equivalent of both English *a* and *one* is a single word, *un(o/a)*. The non-specific/quantifier distinction is not available in Spanish in this structure. Thus, if I tell you I am going shopping for 'un vestido rojo', it could be I mean either non-specifically any red dress or exactly one red dress.

Consider, then, if a Spanish-English bilingual child uses 'one X' as if it is non-specific for number (that is, as if it is 'a X'). This could well arise from an association of *one* in English with *un(o/a)* in Spanish, not because a child cannot tell the difference between one and two. (An interesting example of this in production occurred in a message sent by a French-English bilingual recently to the first author concerning applications for a post. French is structured like Spanish in this regard: 'Please let me know if I have missed one applicant with interest in our group'.)

Other examples abound in the child language literature of differences across languages: Just to give some examples: English makes a distinction between putting things *on* and *in* other things; Korean cross-cuts this by making a distinction between putting things in a tight- versus loose-fit relationship (Bowerman & Choi, 2001). English and similar languages encode the manner of movement in the main verb of a sentence and the path in a preposition (*she hopped across the road, he ran out of the shop*, etc.); many languages encode the path in the main verb and the manner in a separate verb or phrase (Spanish: *cruzó la calle saltando* '(she) crossed the street hopping/jumping'; *salió de la tienda corriendo* '(he) exited the shop running'). These differences have effects on the number of manner verbs available in the two types of languages, on whether speakers pay attention to agents causing movement, on how violent listeners perceive criminals to be, and the like (Choi, 2009; Filipovic, 2010, in press; Slobin 1996, 2009).

For the general purpose of gaining information on a child's conceptual abilities, then, it is clear that either bypassing language in obtaining that information or knowing something about bilingual children's abilities in both of their languages is indispensable.

Language-related purposes of assessment

When we turn to assessment aimed specifically at language, there are again several purposes for which tests are used. On the one hand, one might want to have information on a child's knowledge of the particular language in question. For example, a teacher may wish to set up reading groups according to the children's knowledge of the language, so assessing that knowledge would be helpful. In such a case, assessment of that language alone could serve the immediate purpose.

On the other hand, one may have a broader aim of determining a child's general linguistic ability or of deciphering if a given child may have a language difficulty per se. With monolingual children, a child's performance on any normed language measure can be taken not only as giving information on what the child knows about the particular language tested, but also as giving information on whether this child is having difficulty with language in general – i.e. whether s/he may have a language disability of some sort.

With bilingual children, this use of normed language measures is not warranted, if the child is tested in only one of his/her languages (Pearson *et al.*, 1993, 1995; Peña *et al.*, 2013), and especially if the test is normed on monolingual children. In rare circumstances could a professional test a bilingual child in only one of his/her languages and be confident in drawing inferences about that child's overall language capacity. At a minimum, if a child shows difficulty in one language, that should ideally be followed up with measures in the child's other language to ensure that one has simply not been sampling either a language that the child has had little or less exposure to than his/her peers or linguistic items that the child has simply not been exposed to in the given language. And in the best of possible worlds, information on both of the child's languages would be desirable before one could draw inferences about overall abilities: The best test for whether a bilingual child is having difficulties with language per se is that s/he should have difficulties in both languages (see, e.g. Håkansson *et al.*, 2003; Peña *et al.*, 2013). In the case in which a professional wishes to determine a child's overall language abilities, then, assessing a bilingual child in one language

alone and comparing him/her with norms based on monolingual development is inappropriate. One needs in the very least to take the child's exposure to the language being tested into account, and in the ideal case one
should measure the child's abilities in both his/her languages.

Bilingual Norming

Tests are not always available in both of the child's languages. To use a
single language measure as an indicator of language capacity per se, the professional needs a way of taking into account the child's level of exposure to
each language (e.g. at home and in school). If differential exposure is built into
the norming of a test, this can at least be taken into consideration when determining whether the child falls within or outside the norms for his or her
cohort. If the child falls outside the norm observed in children with similar
language exposure, it may then be taken as a first indication of potential problems. (Such a possibility could then be pursued through further exploration.)

A number of tests have begun providing bilingual norms, alongside monolingual norms, for standardized tests. Some good examples are Brownell (2000a,
2000b) for Spanish-English bilinguals; Munro *et al.* (2005) for Welsh bilinguals;
Verhoeven and Vermeer (1993) for Dutch monolinguals and bilinguals; Munoz-
Sandoval *et al.* (2005) for bilingual abilities in 18 languages; Mattes (1995) for
vocabulary in English in combination with Spanish, French, Italian, or
Vietnamese; and Paradis and Libben (1987) for aphasic individuals (available in
65 languages and 170 language pairs). The BPVS (Dunn *et al.*, 1997) also now
provides norms for bilingual children. And bilingual versions of the CDI are
being developed (see O'Toole, 2013; Ezeizabarrena *et al.*, 2013).

These newer tests typically provide one set of norms for bilingual children (or for children from a certain L1 background learning a given L2, e.g.
Verhoeven & Vermeer, 1993), different from the norms for monolingual children. They, thus, acknowledge that bilingual children's more limited exposure to a language can affect their performance. However, most of these tests
do not distinguish between sub-groups (e.g. those from distinct L1 language
backgrounds or those who are learning only language A at home and language B at school vs. those learning both languages A and B at school, and so
forth). They thus sometimes provide only a very crude measure of a bilingual
child's abilities.

It would be beneficial if a test of a child's linguistic abilities could provide
information on both (a) where the child falls relative to the whole population
(both bilingual and monolingual) of a similar age range and (b) where the
child falls relative to precisely those bilingual children who have similar
exposure to the language, not just in comparison with any bilingual. This
dual-pronged assessment would then provide information on where a given
child stands from the two perspectives – where the child stands in relation

to all children learning the given language, and where the child stands in relation to children with a similar exposure to the language.

We have begun designing such tests for use with bilingual Welsh-English-speaking children. We have normed two versions of our receptive vocabulary test, the *Prawf Geirfa Cymraeg*, one for ages 7 to 11 (Gathercole & Thomas, 2007), the other for 11 to 15 (Gathercole *et al.*, in press), and are similarly developing a version for 2- to 7-year-olds. We are also in the process of norming a picture naming task, receptive grammar tasks, a semantic fluency task, and a productive grammar task in a similar fashion.

Two elements of these tests go beyond the typical norming for such measures. First, one of the primary innovations of the norming is that children's language experience is taken into consideration in conducting analyses of data collected through testing. (For a full account of the design of the *Prawf Geirfa Cymraeg: Fersiwn 7–11*, see Gathercole *et al.*, 2008 and Gathercole & Thomas, 2007.) Most importantly, children are grouped according to the language(s) that their parents speak to them in the home – only or mostly Welsh at home (OWH), only or mostly English at home (OEH), or both Welsh and English at home (WEH). In every analysis we have conducted to date, home language is a significant variable in how children perform. We have therefore incorporated home language as a factor in assigning norms to performance. The second innovation is that each child receives two normed scores, one comparing him/her to the performance of all children at the given age, the other comparing him/her to the performance of children with similar linguistic experience.

For example, the normed version of the *PGC* for 7- to 11-year-olds presents those lexical items that are discriminative of performance across children at the ages tested. Based on the child's responses, s/he receives two sets of norms: an 'Age-Standard Score', which places the child's performance relative to his age-matched peers regardless of home language background, and an 'Age-Year X Home Language Standard Score', which places the child's performance relative to his/her age and year-matched peers from a comparable home language background. Both norms can then be consulted when considering a given bilingual individual child's level of vocabulary.

Table 2.10 provides an example of a blank form that is used for recording each child's performance on our vocabulary measure for the 7- to 11-year-olds. All of the following are included in the explicit score report: the child's age group, year in school, and Home Language group, the child's raw score, and both standardized scores. The form explicitly notes, to provide a constant reminder to the tester and anyone trying to interpret the results, that the 'AGE Standard Score' is 'For comparison with ALL children at this age', and the 'AGE-YEAR X HOME LANGUAGE Standard Score' is 'For comparison ONLY with children at this age and year from the same language background'.

This information together constitutes the child's 'score' on the test. Once the score has been derived, it then requires interpretation. The assessor

Table 2.10 Form for entering raw and standardized scores, *Prawf Geirfa Cymraeg* (Gathercole & Thomas, 2007)

Name	Background details			Raw score	Standardized scores		Interpretation			
	Age	Year	Home language		AGE Standard score	AGE - YEAR X HOME LANGUAGE Standard score	Within normal range	Possible language difficulty	Probable language difficulty	High language ability
					For comparison with ALL children at this age	For comparison ONLY with children at this age and year from same language background				
						Comparison group				

makes a judgment on the best interpretation of the child's abilities, based on the child's age, Home Language, and the standardized scores, and can make a note of that interpretation directly on the form. In every case, all scores should be consulted when evaluating a given child's performance. If both standard scores show either below- or above-normal performance, the evaluator can make decisions confidently on the basis of that performance. However, when the Age-Year X Home Language standard score suggests a different assessment of the child's abilities (below, at, or above the norm) than the general Age-standard score, then further investigation is warranted (See Gathercole *et al.*, 2008, for elaboration).

Norming that takes into account exposure beyond the home language may be necessary in some cases. For example, in a context in which there is a clear demarcation in the language(s) used for instruction in schools (e.g. between schools that teach only through the medium of one of the languages and schools that teach through the medium of both languages), this could be considered as a variable that may be of importance in flagging the type of exposure a given child has to the language(s) in question. Or another example of a potentially important factor is the language(s) prominent in the overall community in which the child is growing up.

This latter factor, in fact, is one that we have found to be crucial for performance among older children on Welsh vocabulary. It has thus been incorporated into our norming for our receptive vocabulary measure for 11- to 15-year-old children in Welsh (Gathercole *et al.*, in press). To be specific, on analysis of the data, we found that, although the community language was not significant in the case of children growing up in OWH and WEH homes, it was significant for 14- and 15-year-olds coming from OEH homes. If OEH children at these ages are living in communities in which 65% or more of the inhabitants are Welsh speakers, their Welsh vocabularies continue to expand beyond the level of OEH children at younger ages. However, if OEH children at these ages are living in communities in which fewer than 65% of the community are Welsh speakers, their Welsh vocabularies do not continue to expand. (At these ages, there are important changes to children's academic choices in school that can have an impact on whether or not they have continuing exposure to Welsh at school. See Thomas *et al.*, 2013.) Our normed version of the test, therefore, reflects the fact that this important exposure variable needs to be taken into consideration in evaluating the Welsh vocabulary performance of OEH children at these ages.

Discussion

This chapter examines assessment of language proficiency in bilingual children and attempts to spell out how bilingual children's linguistic development in their two languages advances at a different pace from linguistic development in monolingual children, and to explore the extent to which children's performance in one language can be taken as indicative of their knowledge of the other language. The data presented above make it clear that a child's abilities in one language have no necessary relationship with his/her abilities in the other language, and, therefore, that one cannot assess children's performance in one language to gain insight into their performance in the other, nor into their overall linguistic abilities.

Standardized assessment measures for language are simply tools for determining whether a given child is developing as one might expect, given his/her circumstances. They are nothing more and nothing less. A given child can be viewed as a member of a large age-matched group, or, alternatively, as a member of a smaller group that share similar experiences and exposure to language. Because standardized language measures, and vocabulary measures in particular, are interpreted as indicating much more than language development (as outlined above), it is imperative that test developers and test users take the steps necessary to ensure that such assessment measures accurately reflect bilingual children's abilities, as practitioners and researchers have argued over the years.

The model described in this chapter is one attempt at accomplishing that goal. It proposes that adequate language measures for bilingual children must take (at least) children's language exposure into account in order to provide an appropriate assessment of their linguistic abilities. Given the importance of standardized tests and their wide use for a variety of purposes, adoption of a model that explicitly takes account of the facts of bilingual development is warranted. Until such tests are available, interpretation of language tests (and any other tests that rely on language for proper performance – i.e. most tests) should proceed with extreme caution.

Acknowledgments and Author Contributions

This work is supported in part by WAG grants on 'Standardized measures for the assessment of Welsh' and on 'Continued development of standardized measures for the assessment of Welsh' (Gathercole PI, Thomas co-investigator), ESRC grant RES-062-23-0175 (Gathercole PI, Thomas co-investigator), and ESRC/WAG/HEFCW grant RES-535-30-0061 (Deuchar, Gathercole, Baker, & Thierry). We are grateful to the schools, teachers, parents, children and adults who participated in these studies. Without their generous cooperation, this work could not be accomplished. This work reflects a collaboration across many levels of research. Gathercole headed the projects involved and analyzed and wrote the materials presented here. Thomas collaborated on the design of the stimuli and tests and in the overall operation of the studies. Roberts, Hughes, and Hughes were researchers on the projects and helped prepare the tests, administered tests to participants and entered data to be analyzed. We are also grateful to Lowri Cunnington, Kelly Davis, Sinead Dolan, Katie

Gibbins, Craig Harris, Leah Jones, Cheryl King, Siwan Long, Hannah Perryman, Cynog Prys, Mirain Rhys, Kathryn Sharp, Nestor Viñas Guasch and Nia Young, who collected a portion of the data in conjunction with other projects, with their final year projects, or as paid hourly assistants.

References

Bowerman, M. (1996a) Learning how to structure space for language: A crosslinguistic perspective. In P. Bloom, M.A. Peterson, L. Nadel and M.F. Garrett (eds) *Language and Space* (pp. 385–436). Cambridge, MA: MIT Press.

Bowerman, M. (1996b) The origins of children's spatial semantic categories: Cognitive versus linguistic determinants. In J.J. Gumperz and S.C. Levinson (eds) *Rethinking Linguistic Relativity* (pp. 145–176). Cambridge: Cambridge University Press.

Bowerman, M. and Choi, S. (2001) Shaping meanings for language: Universal and language-specific in the acquisition of spatial semantic categories. In M. Bowerman and S.C. Levinson (eds) *Language Acquisition and Conceptual Development* (pp. 475–511). Cambridge: Cambridge University Press.

Brownell, R. (2000a) *Expressive One-Word Picture Vocabulary Test: Spanish-Bilingual Edition.* Novato, CA: Academic Therapy Publications.

Brownell, R. (2000b) *Receptive One-Word Picture Vocabulary Test: Spanish-Bilingual Edition.* Novato, CA: Academic Therapy Publications.

Choi, S. (2009) Typological differences in syntactic expressions of path and causation. In V.C.M. Gathercole (ed.) *Routes to Language: Studies in Honor of Melissa Bowerman* (pp. 169–194). N.Y.: Psychology Press.

Cobo-Lewis, A., Pearson, B., Eilers, R. and Umbel, V. (2002a) Bilinguals' oral and written skills in Spanish: A multi-factor study of standardized test outcomes. In D.K. Oller and R. Eilers (eds) *Language and Literacy in Bilingual Children* (pp. 98–117). Clevedon: Multilingual Matters.

Cobo-Lewis, A., Pearson, B., Eilers, R. and Umbel, V. (2002b) Effects of bilingualism and bilingual education on oral and written English skills: A multifactor study of standardized test outcomes. In D.K. Oller and R. Eilers (eds) *Language and Literacy in Bilingual Children* (pp. 43–63). Clevedon: Multilingual Matters.

Cohen, C. (2006) The effect of language experiences on oral proficiency. *Presented at Language Acquisition and Bilingualism: Consequences for a Multilingual Society*, Toronto, May 4–7.

Dijkstra, T. and van Hell, J.G. (2003) Testing the Language Mode Hypothesis using trilinguals. *International Journal of Bilingual Education and Bilingualism* 6, 2–16.

Dijkstra, T. and Van Heuven, W.J.B. (1998) The BIA-model and bilingual word recognition. In J. Grainger and A. Jacobs (eds) *Localist Connectionist Approaches to Human Cognition* (pp. 189–225). Hillsdale, NJ: Erlbaum.

Döpke, S. (1998) Competing language structures: The acquisition of verb placement by bilingual German-English children. *Journal of Child Language* 25, 555–584.

Döpke, S. (2000) The interplay between language-specific development and crosslinguistic influence. In S. Döpke (ed.) *Cross-linguistic Structures in Simultaneous Bilingualism.* Amsterdam: Benjamins.

Dunn, L.M., Dunn, L.M., Whetton, C. and Burley, J. (1997) *The British Picture Vocabulary Scale: Second Edition.* NFER-NELSON.

Ellis, N.C., O'Dochartaigh, C., Hicks, W., Morgan, M. and Laporte, N. (2001) Cronfa Electroneg o Gymraeg/ A 1 million word lexical database and frequency count for Welsh. University of Wales Bangor: School of Psychology. http://www.bangor.ac.uk/ar/cb/ceg/ceg_cym.html

Elston-Güttler, K. and Williams, J.N. (2008) L1 polysemy affects L2 meaning interpretation: Evidence for L1 concepts active during L2 reading. *Second Language Research* 24, 167–187.

Ezeizabarrena, M-J., Barnes, J., García, I., Barreña, A. and Almgren, M. (2013). Using parental report assessment for bilingual preschoolers: The Basque experience. In V.C.M. Gathercole (ed.) *Solutions for the Assessment of Bilinguals* (pp. 57–80). Bristol: Multilingual Matters.

Filipovic, L. (2010) Thinking and speaking about motion: Universal vs. language-specific effects. In G. Marotta, A. Lenci, L. Meini and F. Rovai (eds) *Space in Language: Proceedings of the Pisa International Conference* (pp. 235–248). University of Pisa.

Filipovic, L. (2011) Speaking and remembering in one or two languages: Bilingual vs. monolingual lexicalization and memory for motion events. *International Journal of Bilingualism* 15 (4), 466–485.

Gathercole, V.C.M. (2009a) Developmental constructivist perspective of interaction in 2L1 acquisition. In Colloquium on 'Crosslinguistic influence on different grammatical domains in bilingual first language acquisition', 7th International Symposium on Bilingualism, July 8–11, 2009, Utrecht, The Netherlands.

Gathercole, V.C.M. (2009b) 'It was so much fun. It was 20 fun!' Cognitive and linguistic invitations to the development of scalar predicates. In V.C.M. Gathercole (ed.) *Routes to Language: Studies in Honor of Melissa Bowerman* (pp. 319–443). N.Y.: Psychology Press, Taylor and Francis.

Gathercole, V.C.M. (2010) Bilingual children: Language and assessment issues for educators. In K. Littleton, C. Wood and J. Kleine Staarman (eds) *Handbook of Psychology in Education* (pp. 713–748). Bingley: Emerald Group.

Gathercole, V.C.M. and Moawad, R. (2010) Semantic interaction in early and late bilinguals: All words are not created equally. *Bilingualism: Language and Cognition* 13 (4), 1–22.

Gathercole, V.C.M., Pérez-Tattam, R. and Stadthagen-González, H. (in press) Bilingual construction of two systems: To interact or not to interact? In E.M. Thomas and I. Mennen (eds) *Unravelling Bilingualism: A Cross-disciplinary Perspective*. Bristol: Multilingual Matters.

Gathercole, V.C.M., Stadthagen-González, H., Pérez-Tattam, R. and Yavas, F. (2011) Semantic organization in bilinguals. Paper presented in Colloquium on dynamic lexical interaction of L1 and L2. International Symposium on Bilingualism 8, Oslo. June 15–18, 2011.

Gathercole, V.C.M. and Thomas, E.M. (2007) *Prawf Geirfa Cymraeg, Fersiwn 7–11.* (Welsh Vocabulary Test, Version 7–11). 2007. www.pgc.bangor.ac.uk.

Gathercole, V.C.M. and Thomas, E.M. (2009) Bilingual first-language development: Dominant language takeover, threatened minority language take-up. *Bilingualism: Language and Cognition* 12, 213–237.

Gathercole, V.C.M., Thomas, E.M. and Hughes, E.K. (2008) Designing a normed receptive vocabulary test for bilingual populations: A model from Welsh. *International Journal of Bilingual Education and Bilingualism* 11 (6), 678–720.

Gathercole, V.C.M., Thomas, E.M. and Hughes, E.K. (in press) *Prawf Geirfa Cymraeg, Fersiwn 11–15.* (Welsh Vocabulary Test, Version 11–15).

Gathercole, V.C.M., Thomas, E.M., Jones, L., Viñas Guasch, N., Young, N. and Hughes, E.K. (2010) Cognitive effects of bilingualism: Digging deeper for the contributions of language dominance, linguistic knowledge, socioeconomic status, and cognitive abilities. *International Journal of Bilingual Education and Bilingualism* 13 (5), 617–664.

Gathercole, V.C.M., Thomas, E.M., Young, N., Viñas Guasch, N., Hughes, E.K. and Jones, L. (resubmitted). Language dominance and executive function in bilinguals: Evidence from card sorting tasks.

Grosjean, F. (1998) Studying bilinguals: Methodological and conceptual issues. *Bilingualism: Language and Cognition* 1, 131–149.

Grosjean, F. (2001) The bilingual's language modes. In J.L. Nicol (ed.) *One Mind, Two Languages: Bilingual Language Processing* (pp. 1–22). Oxford: Blackwell.

Håkansson, G., Salameh, E-K. and Nettelbladt, U. (2003) Measuring language development in bilingual children: Swedish-Arabic children with and without language impairment. *Linguistics* 41–2, 255–288.

Hoff, E., Core, C., Place, S., Rumiche, R., Señor, M. and Parra, M. (2012) Dual language exposure and early bilingual development. *Journal of Child Language* 39 (1), 1–27.

Hulk, A. and Müller, N. (2000) Bilingual first language acquisition at the interface between syntax and pragmatics. *Bilingualism: Language and Cognition* 3 (3), 227–244.

Malt, B.C., Sloman, S.A. and Gennari, S.P. (2003) Universality and language specificity in object naming. *Journal of Memory and Language* 29, 20–42.

Mattes, L.J. (1995) *Bilingual Vocabulary Assessment Measure.* Oceanside, CA: Academic Communication Associates.

McCarthy, D. (1972) *McCarthy Scales of Children's Abilities.* San Antonio: Harcourt Assessment.

Meisel, J. (1989) Early differentiation of languages in bilingual children. In K. Hyltenstam and L. Obler (eds) *Bilingualism Across the Lifespan: Aspects of Acquisition, Maturity, and Loss* (pp. 13–40). Cambridge: Cambridge University Press.

Meisel, J. (2001) The simultaneous acquisition of two first languages: Early differentiation and subsequent development of grammars. In J. Cenoz and F. Genesee (eds) *Trends in Bilingual Acquisition* (pp. 11–41). Amsterdam: Benjamins.

Munoz-Sandoval, A.F., Cummins, J., Alvarado, G. and Ruef, M.L. (2005) *Bilingual Verbal Ability Test.* Scarborough, ON: Thomson Nelson.

Munro, S., Ball, M., Müller, N., Duckworth, M. and Lyddy, F. (2005) Phonological acquisition in Welsh-English bilingual children. *Journal of Multilingual Communication Disorders* 3 (1), 24 – 49.

Oller, D.K. (2005) The distributed characteristic in bilingual learning. In J. Cohen, K. McAlister, K. Rolstad and J. MacSwan (eds) *ISB4: Proceedings of the 4th International Symposium on Bilingualism* (pp. 1744–1749). Somerville, MA: Cascadilla Press.

Oller, D.K. and Pearson, B.Z. (2002) Assessing the effects of bilingualism: A background. In D.K. Oller and R.E. Eilers (eds) *Language and Literacy in Bilingual Children* (pp. 3–21). Clevedon: Multilingual Matters.

O'Toole, C. (2013) Using parent report to assess bilingual vocabulary acquisition: A model from Irish. In V.C.M. Gathercole (ed.) *Solutions for the Assessment of Bilinguals* (pp. 81–102). Bristol: Multilingual Matters.

Paradis, J. and Genesee, F. (1996) Syntactic acquisition: Autonomous or interdependent? *Studies in Second Language Acquisition* 18, 1–25.

Paradis, M. and Libben, G. (1987) *The Assessment of Bilingual Aphasia.* Hillsdale, NJ: Erlbaum.

Pavlenko, A. (ed.) (2009) *The Bilingual Mental Lexicon: Interdisciplinary Approaches.* Bristol: Multilingual Matters.

Pearson, B.Z. and Fernández, S. (1994) Patterns of interaction in the lexical growth in two languages of bilingual infants and toddlers. *Language Learning* 44, 617–653.

Pearson, B.Z., Fernández, S. and Oller, D.K. (1993) Lexical development in bilingual infants and toddlers: Comparison to monolingual norms. *Language Learning* 43, 93–120.

Pearson, B.Z., Fernández, S. and Oller, D.K. (1995) Cross-language synonyms in the lexicons of bilingual infants: One language or two? *Journal of Child Language* 22, 345–368.

Peña, E.D., Bedore, L.M. and Fiestas, C. (2013) Development of bilingual semantic norms: Can two be one? In V.C.M. Gathercole (ed.) *Solutions for the Assessment of Bilinguals* (pp. 103–124). Bristol: Multilingual Matters.

Place, S. and Hoff, E. (2011) Properties of dual language exposure that influence 2-year-olds' bilingual proficiency. *Child Development* 82 (6), 1834–1849.

Raven, J., Raven, J.C. and Court, J.H. (2004) *Manual for Raven's Progressive Matrices and Vocabulary Scales*. San Antonio, TX: Pearson Assessment.

Reynell, J. (1987) *Reynell Developmental Language Scales: Welsh Adaptation*. NFER-NELSON.

Slobin, D.I. (1996) From 'thought and language' to 'thinking for speaking'. In J.J. Gumperz and S.C. Levinson (eds) *Rethinking Linguistic Relativity* (pp. 70–96). Cambridge: Cambridge University Press.

Slobin, D.I. (2009) Relations between paths of motion and paths of vision: A crosslinguistic and developmental exploration. In V.C.M. Gathercole (ed.) *Routes to Language: Studies in Honor of Melissa Bowerman* (pp. 197–222). NY: Psychology Press.

Thomas, E.M. and Gathercole, V.C.M. (2007) Children's productive command of grammatical gender and mutation in Welsh: An alternative to rule-based learning. *First Language* 27, 251–278.

Thomas, E.M., Gathercole, V.C.M. and Hughes, E.K. (2013) Sociolinguistic influences on the linguistic achievement of bilinguals: Issues for the assessment of minority language competence. In V.C.M. Gathercole (ed.) *Solutions for the Assessment of Bilinguals* (pp. 175–193). Bristol: Multilingual Matters.

Umbel, V.M., Pearson, B.Z., Fernández, M.C. and Oller, D.K. (1992) Measuring bilingual children's receptive vocabularies. *Child Development* 63, 1012–1020.

Verhoeven, L. and Vermeer, A. (1993) *Taaltoets Allochtone Kinderen Bovenbouw* [Language Tests for Minority Children]. Tilburg, The Netherlands: Zwijsen.

3 Assessment of Language Abilities in Sequential Bilingual Children: The Potential of Sentence Imitation Tasks

Shula Chiat, Sharon Armon-Lotem, Theodoros Marinis, Kamila Polišenská, Penny Roy and Belinda Seeff-Gabriel

Sentence repetition tasks are increasingly recognised as a useful clinical tool for assessing children's language skills, diagnosing language impairment and determining targets for intervention. They are quick to administer, can be carefully targeted to elicit specific sentence structures and are particularly informative about children's lexical and morphosyntactic knowledge. This chapter explores the theoretical potential of sentence repetition for assessment of sequential bilingual children, and presents three studies comparing performance of sequential bilingual children with monolingual children's performance on standardized sentence repetition tests in Hebrew (children with L1 Russian, age 5–7 years, and L1 English, age 4½–6½ years), German (children with L1 Russian, age 4–7 years) and English (children with L1 Turkish, age 6–9 years). Results differed across studies: the distribution of children in the Hebrew studies was in line with the monolingual norms, while the majority of children in the English-Turkish study scored in a range that would be deemed impaired for monolingual children, and performance in the German-Russian study fell between these extremes. Analyses of performance within studies revealed similar discrepancies in effects of children's exposure to L2, with significant effects of Age of Onset in the Hebrew-Russian and Hebrew-English groups and some indication of Length of Exposure effects, but no effects of either factor in the English-Turkish group. Multiple differences between these studies preclude direct inferences about the reasons for these different results: studies differed in content, methods and scoring of sentence repetition tests, and in ages, languages, language exposure and socioeconomic status of participants. It is possible that socioeconomic differences are associated with differences in language experience that are equally or more important than onset and length of exposure. Collectively, these studies demonstrate that sentence repetition provides a method for assessing children's proficiency in their L2, but that the use of sentence repetition in clinical assessment requires caution unless norms are available for the child's bilingual community. As a next step, it is proposed that sentence repetition tests using early-acquired vocabulary and targeting aspects of sentence structure known to be difficult for monolingual children with language impairments should be developed in different target languages. This will allow us to explore further the factors that influence attainment of basic morphosyntax in sequential bilingual children, and the point at which sentence repetition, as an assessment of morphosyntax, can help to identify children requiring clinical intervention.

The challenges of assessing language and identifying language impairment in bilingual children are all too familiar to clinicians. How can the child's language be meaningfully assessed if there are no standardized assessments of the child's L1, and performance on L2 assessments may reflect limited exposure to L2 rather than a developmental deficit? In this chapter, we make a case for the potential contribution of verbal imitation tasks – and more specifically sentence imitation tasks – in addressing these challenges. In the first part of the chapter, we review evidence that verbal imitation is highly informative about children's expressive language and differentiates children with SLI from typically developing children in diverse and typologically different languages. We then consider the role of language knowledge and experience in repetition tasks based on studies revealing the influence of linguistic and environmental factors on children's performance. The second part of the chapter presents studies of sentence imitation in four groups of children with different L1–L2 combinations. Based on theoretical and empirical evidence presented in the chapter, we put forward a multilingual agenda for developing and evaluating sentence imitation tasks to assess core language abilities in children's L2.

Verbal Imitation as Evidence of Language Abilities and Deficits

In the early days of child language research, children's ability to imitate sentences attracted cursory attention, reflecting the theoretical perspective of the day. It was observed that children imitated 'within their system', be it phonological (Smith, 1973) or syntactic (Brown, 1973). However, this served merely to supplement the rationalist argument that language could not be acquired by imitation of input, with empirical evidence that imitating the input does not help children achieve the adult model or attain the adult system. A few early investigations explored relations between imitation, comprehension and production of language in naturalistic and experimental situations (e.g. Fraser *et al.*, 1963), but pursuit of imitation in child language research and the impact on clinical assessment were limited. Exceptionally, the Carrow Elicited Language Inventory (Carrow, 1974) assesses sentence imitation in its own right, but there is little evidence of its use in clinical assessment or research.

When interest in children's ability to imitate surfaced again, some two decades later, it was in the very different guise of the nonword repetition task, which has come to occupy a privileged position in research on Specific Language Impairment (SLI) and developmental dyslexia. The nonword repetition test was originally developed by Gathercole and Baddeley (1989) as a relatively pure measure of phonological short-term memory (STM). The rationale for using nonwords as stimuli was that this would minimise the contribution of children's knowledge to their performance. The finding that nonword repetition performance related to children's wider language and reading abilities could then be advanced as evidence for the crucial contribution of phonological memory to the development of these complex skills.

The broad findings on nonword repetition for monolingual children are not in doubt. They have been replicated in a raft of studies reporting significant differences between typically developing monolingual children and children with SLI in English (see Coady & Evans, 2008; Gathercole, 2006; and Graf Estes *et al.*, 2007 for overviews). Group differences have been reported for children at different ages and in different languages including Swedish (Sahlén *et al.*, 1999), Italian (Casalini *et al.*, 2007) and Spanish (Girbau & Schwartz, 2007). Indeed, the consistency of findings has led to the proposal that nonword repetition may serve as a clinical marker for SLI. To date, only one study has gone against the tide of crosslinguistic evidence, reporting no difference between children with and without SLI in Cantonese (Stokes *et al.*, 2006).

Although not as prolifically researched as nonword repetition, sentence repetition has been gaining attention as another possible marker of SLI in monolingual children. Clinical assessments of language often include a sentence recall subtest, as in the case of the Clinical Evaluation of Language Fundamentals (CELF; Semel *et al.*, 1994; Wiig *et al.*, 1992) and the Test of Language Development (TOLD; Newcomer & Hammill, 1997). Most studies of sentence repetition in English have employed the Sentence Recall subtest of the CELF, and have found significant differences between children with SLI and typically developing (TD) peers (Bishop *et al.*, 2009; Conti-Ramsden *et al.*, 2001). In a comparison of four candidate clinical markers, Conti-Ramsden *et al.* found that Sentence Recall achieved the best combination of sensitivity and specificity. Studies using other sets of sentence stimuli have found significant differences between typically developing (TD), SLI, and other clinical groups (Redmond, 2005; Redmond *et al.*, 2011; Riches *et al.*, 2010; Willis & Gathercole, 2001). Seeff-Gabriel *et al.* (2010) report on a sentence repetition test designed for children with severe speech difficulties. This test also yielded significant differences between children with SLI and TD peers, and Seeff-Gabriel *et al.* demonstrated its capacity to identify intact morphosyntactic abilities in children with unintelligible speech whose expressive language defied assessment using other methods. In the case of sentence repetition, even the Cantonese data fall into line: Stokes *et al.* report significant differences between their groups of children with SLI and age-matched TD peers on a test of sentence repetition in Cantonese.

The Rationale for Exploring Sentence Repetition Tasks as a Method for Assessing Children in Their L2

Repetition tasks have a number of advantages that make them particularly attractive for L2 assessment. They are quick and easy to administer; in contrast to most language elicitation tasks, linguistic targets are explicit and precisely specified; and they yield clear quantitative and qualitative results. As targets are known and consistent, we can readily compare levels of performance and patterns of errors across children, making it easy to track children's progress in relation to typical performance whether in L1 or L2. These strengths are clearly exemplified by sentence repetition tasks. If carefully constructed, a set of 20 to 40 sentences allows sampling of a rich and representative range of sentence structures, which it would be difficult, if not impossible, to elicit through a sentence production task or collection of spontaneous language data. The Sentence Imitation Test (SIT; Seeff-Gabriel *et al.*, 2008), for example, contains a comprehensive range of simple sentence structures sampling a comprehensive range of function words in English. This provides information about the aspects of sentences that children find difficult, which is very useful for therapy planning.

Alongside these general advantages, repetition tasks have a special role to play in L2 assessment, to the extent that they can be shown to be less affected by exposure and experience, which are known to be limited in L2. In the next section, we consider the ways in which linguistic characteristics of the stimulus materials affect children's repetition performance, revealing the benefits of language knowledge and by implication language experience. We then consider the effects of environmental differences on sentence repetition as evidenced by the performance of children from socially disadvantaged backgrounds who may be at risk of language disadvantage in their L1.

The Contribution of Language-Specific Knowledge to Sentence Repetition

It is now widely accepted that even nonword repetition, which was originally proposed as a 'pure' measure of phonological short-term memory, is subject to the familiarity of targets (Gathercole, 2006). All nonword repetition tests contain items that are consistent with the phonetics of the target language, being made up of consonants and vowels that occur in that language. However, tests vary substantially in word-likeness of their nonwords (and even within tests, individual items may be more or less word-like): they may be characterised by more or less typical prosodic structure, more or less frequent phonotactic sequences, and may or may not contain morphemes of the language. All these factors turn out to influence children's nonword repetition performance (see Gathercole, 2006), demonstrating the effects of phonetic, phonological and morphological knowledge on the perception, storage and production of novel phonological forms. Nevertheless, influences on nonword repetition are clearly circumscribed compared with repetition of sentences, which open the floodgates to potential sources of support from language-specific knowledge. Sentences contain real words comprising fixed phonological forms with specific meanings, and these are combined according to the syntax and morphosyntax of the language to convey meaningful relations. Given the effects of phonology and morphology on nonword repetition, we might expect sentence repetition to be even more affected by familiarity with structures of the language.

A recent study by Polišenská (2011, under review) set out to address this issue by investigating the extent to which different types of language knowledge influence children's short-term memory span for sequences of words. Fifty typically developing Czech children and 50 typically developing English children aged 4 to 6 years participated in this study. The children were presented with blocks of successively longer sequences of words in different linguistic conditions, in order to determine their maximum span in each condition. The different conditions systematically varied syntactic, semantic, lexical and prosodic properties, as illustrated by the following examples of four-item length:

A	Well-formed sentence	*I hurt my knee*
B	Well-formed sentence with list prosody	*I, hurt, my, knee*
C	Semantically implausible sentence	*I dug my tea*
D	Pseudosentence with all lexical items replaced by nonwords	/ɔɪ vɜt kaɪ ri/
E	Syntactically ill-formed pseudosentence with sentence prosody	*Hurt my I knee*
F	Pseudosentence with content words replaced by nonwords	*I* /vɜt/ *my* /ri/
G	Pseudosentence with function words replaced by nonwords	/ɔɪ/ *hurt* /kaɪ/ *knee*

Comparison of conditions revealed the effect of each factor on immediate repetition performance. Prosodic structure (condition A vs B) had a significant effect, increasing memory span from a mean of 7.5 to 8.01 words in English and 7 to 7.58 in Czech, with a mean difference of 0.51 and 0.58, respectively. Semantic plausibility (condition A vs C) had a similar effect, increasing memory span from a mean of 7.05 to 8.01 words in English and 6.74 to 7.58 in Czech, a mean difference of 0.96 and 0.84, respectively. Familiarity of syntax and lexical items, however, produced the most notable effects. Lexical familiarity (condition A vs D), which brings with it morphosyntactic relations, dramatically increased memory span from a mean of 2.84 to 8.01 words in English and 2.54 to 7.58 in Czech, a mean difference of 5.17 and 5.04, respectively. Effects of morphosyntactic structure alone (condition A vs E) were almost as dramatic, with memory span increasing from a mean of 4.35 to 8.01 words in English and 3.9 to 7.58 in Czech, a mean difference of 3.66 and 3.68, respectively. Although the freer word order of Czech reduced possibilities for word order violations in the syntactically ill-formed condition, the effects of such violations were similar. Furthermore, despite its more limited repertoire of function words and greater reliance on inflections (which were not manipulated in this study), Czech showed a similar advantage for sentences containing real function words combined with nonwords in content word slots (condition F), compared with sentences containing real content words combined with nonwords in function word slots (condition G). The difference between spans in these two conditions was statistically significant in both languages: 1.34 words in English and 0.97 in Czech. It seems that the form and distribution of closed class words, once acquired, are extremely robust and support immediate recall of verbal material.

Polišenská's findings demonstrate that sentence repetition draws on all aspects of sentence knowledge, but most distinctively on knowledge of syntax and morphosyntax. The implication is that children's repetition of simple sentences with familiar vocabulary is most informative about children's syntactic and morphosyntactic knowledge: their familiarity with words and the morphosyntactic devices that mark relations between these. Studies of early sentence repetition support this conclusion. In an investigation of sentence repetition in Italian TD preschoolers, Devescovi and Caselli (2007) found that omission of articles, prepositions and modifiers decreased between 2;0 and 2;6, and after 3 years of age, 'omissions of free function words practically disappeared' (p. 188). Grammatical morphemes are known to be a particular challenge for children with language impairment, and persisting difficulties with grammatical morphology are frequently seen as a hallmark of SLI (Leonard, 1998). If simple sentence repetition is an effective test of grammatical morphology, it is unsurprising that it is a strong candidate for assessing children's language and identifying SLI (see above).

Effects of Variation in Language Experience on Sentence Imitation in L1

Whereas the effects of knowledge and therefore experience of a specific language on repetition are clear, the effects of variations in experience *within* a language have received relatively little attention. Indeed, a key motivation for using nonword repetition as a clinical indicator is the claim that it tests processing skills that are relatively immune to prior knowledge and experience and therefore less biased against children from minority or disadvantaged backgrounds (Campbell *et al.*, 1997; Dollaghan & Campbell, 1998; Roy & Chiat, 2004). Accordingly, Campbell *et al.* found no difference between groups of first-graders from majority (White) and minority (primarily African American) backgrounds on a nonword repetition test. Engel *et al.* (2008) compared nonword repetition performance in 6- to 7-year-old Brazilian children attending public and private schools. The groups were distinguished in terms of care-giver education, professional status, and income. They were found to differ on traditional measures of receptive and expressive language, but not on nonword repetition. The standardisation sample for the Early Repetition Battery (ERB; Seeff-Gabriel *et al.*, 2008) showed very limited effects of socioeconomic status (SES) on the two repetition tests that make up the Battery: the Preschool Repetition Test (PSRep) and Sentence Imitation Test (SIT). Most notably, no significant effect was found for the key measures on the SIT: the number of content words and number of function words repeated correctly.

Based on these findings and others' evidence on nonword repetition in older children, Roy and Chiat (2013) hypothesised that measures of verbal repetition might offer a key to cracking the well-recognised problem of differentiating limitations in language owing to language disorder from limitations due to disadvantage. It was predicted that the distribution of performance on the PSRep and SIT in children from low SES backgrounds would be normal, in contrast to the downward shift in their scores on standard language measures. This hypothesis was investigated in a study of 387 children aged 3½ to 5 years, 219 attending nurseries/schools in Barking and Dagenham, a London borough with a high level of socioeconomic disadvantage, and 168 attending nurseries/schools in mid-to-high SES areas. The results were initially surprising: contrary to previous findings, the low and mid-to-high SES groups differed significantly on these tests, and the low SES group showed a clear deviation from the expected distribution. In the case of the SIT, 26.9% of the low SES children's function word scores fell more than 1 SD below the mean, including 4.1% below −2 SDs. The skewing was even more marked for 'whole sentence correct' scores, with 31.5% of the low SES children more than 1 SD below the mean, including 7.8% below −2 SDs. Further analysis of performance according to age uncovered possible reasons for this unexpected finding, with important implications for the role of experience in verbal repetition. When the data were analysed by 6-month age bands, a cross-sectional developmental trajectory emerged: by age 4 ½ to 5, the gap between the expected and observed distribution of performance in the low SES group had narrowed and in some cases closed. Function word scores below −1 SD were down to 8.2%, including only 1.4% below −2 SDs, although scores for 'whole sentence correct' still found 20.6% of children below −1 SD. In contrast to the changes observed in the low SES group, the distribution in the mid-to-high SES group was stable across ages, with no children scoring below −2 SDs on either of the SIT measures, and over 95% performing within the normal range on both.

How, however, does this evidence square with the evidence that repetition skills are free of SES effects? The subtle evidence of linguistic influences on repetition performance observed in the Polišenská study may supply the missing piece. If detailed knowledge of lexical phonology and morphosyntax contributes to repetition performance, we might expect performance to vary with levels of experience even in L1. Given the lack of effects of SES in previous studies, it seems that variation in exposure for the range of SES groups compared in these studies is not sufficient to affect the emergence of core phonological and morphosyntactic knowledge, and/or the threshold for attaining this knowledge is relatively low (supported by the ERB standardisation results). The reduced performance in the Barking and Dagenham group, however, together with the catch-up in their first year of school, strongly suggests that prior to school this group's language experience was unusually limited, affecting the deployment of core skills and acquisition of core phonological and morphosyntactic knowledge.

Implications for the Investigation of Sentence Repetition Tasks as a Method for Assessing Children in Their L2

We started this chapter by arguing that sentence repetition is an efficient and informative method for assessing children's language ability, and is therefore worth exploring as a method for L2 assessment. We have now seen that sentence repetition draws on language knowledge, particularly lexical and morphosyntactic knowledge, and is affected by extreme differences in social experience. This finding might lead us to conclude that sentence repetition is not after all a particularly useful avenue to explore for assessment of L2 children. As these children are known to have late and/or reduced exposure to the language, how do we know whether a shortfall in sentence repetition performance is attributable to limited experience or to disorder? Our in-depth consideration of influences on sentence repetition has brought us back to the paradox of L2 assessment: the more a test draws on language-specific skills, the better it differentiates children with and without impairment; but the more it draws on language-specific skills, the more it depends on language experience that may be lacking in L2 children. Accordingly, sentence repetition is more clinically informative than nonword repetition using word-like items, which is in turn more informative than nonword repetition using non-word-like items (Archibald & Gathercole, 2006), but this advantage is counterbalanced by greater dependence on linguistic knowledge and therefore experience. Given the unavoidable trade-off between the two ideals for L2 assessment – optimal differentiation of children with language impairment and minimal reliance on language experience – sentence repetition may still have a special role to play. The potential for comprehensive and controlled sampling of targets affords precise and informative measurement of performance; this in turn affords detailed comparison between groups and investigation of the ways in which between-group factors (such as amount and nature of exposure to L2, linguistic characteristics of L1 and L2) affect performance.

The Importance of Test Targets and Scoring

The impact of experience on a sentence repetition test will vary according to the demands it makes on language-specific knowledge and according to the criteria for scoring responses. As we saw with Polišenská's study, repetition of simple sentences is particularly subject to knowledge of lexical phonology, word order, and more specifically, the form and position of function words. In line with this, studies reported by Devescovi and Caselli (2007) and Seeff-Gabriel et al. (2010) revealed that measures of function words are particularly informative about language abilities in typically developing children and children with SLI. In considering the potential of sentence repetition for L2 assessment and the experience required to achieve L1 levels of performance, it will therefore be important to consider test content and how this is scored. In the most widely used measures of sentence repetition in English, the Sentence Recall subtests of the preschool and school-age Clinical Evaluation of Language Fundamentals (CELF; Semel *et al.*, 1994; Wiig *et al.*, 1992), targets vary in syntactic structure and become progressively more complex, but syntax is not systematically manipulated (see section on Turkish-English study below for examples).

In contrast to the Test of Language Development (TOLD; Newcomer & Hammill, 1997), which scores whole responses as right or wrong, CELF uses a more discriminating measure, scoring each response according to the number of errors made. As is clear from research findings, this scoring method is sensitive to group differences. However, the unspecified nature of the targets and purely quantitative scoring provide no information about the source of a child's difficulties or the nature of their errors.

Tests that systematically manipulate stimuli and/or employ more qualitative scoring methods are more informative about group differences. Riches *et al.* (2010), for example, manipulated the syntactic structure of sentences involving long-distance dependencies and employed a sensitive measure for scoring that took account of distance between the target sentence and the response. Using this scoring method, quantitative and qualitative differences were found between a group of adolescents with autism spectrum disorders plus language difficulties and a group with SLI. The SIT (Seeff-Gabriel *et al.*, 2008) was specifically designed to assess morphosyntax in preschool children. This consists of 27 simple sentences that increase in length and complexity. Responses are scored in terms of number of content (open class) words, function (closed class) words and inflections repeated correctly. Each of these broad morphosyntactic classes can be broken down further into specific syntactic categories such as prepositions, auxiliary verbs and pronouns.

The Cantonese sentence repetition test developed by Stokes *et al.* (2006) targeted two morphosyntactic structures, aspect and passive, and employed four scoring methods. Three were purely quantitative, whereas one scored 'core elements' of the target structures. Following findings on function words in English and Italian, we might expect the 'core element' score to be most discriminating and informative. Instead, Stokes *et al.* found that the CELF method of scoring sentences according to number of errors per sentence was the most effective in distinguishing children with and without SLI. It is not immediately obvious why scoring 'core elements' in Cantonese was less discriminating. This may reflect prosodic, semantic, and/or syntactic characteristics of the 'core elements' in Cantonese (as compared with characteristics of grammatical markers in English and Italian). Further insights into patterns of sentence repetition performance in Cantonese await detailed consideration of morphosyntactic categories and relations and the forms that express these, together with evidence of repetition performance on these in TD children and children with SLI.

The Cantonese data provide a salutary reminder that test content will reflect morphosyntactic characteristics of the languages tested, which can vary considerably, and these may have effects on profiles of performance in different groups (typically and atypically developing, L1 and L2) and implications for clinical diagnosis. In the case of L2 children, linguistic characteristics of the L1 may also affect profiles of repetition performance in the L2. Considering this complex constellation of potential influences, any generalisations about the use of sentence repetition in L2 assessment will require comparisons across different and typologically diverse L1–L2 combinations (Gathercole, 2010), as well as variations in children's exposure to each language.

In the following sections of this chapter, we present exploratory investigations of L2 performance on existing sentence repetition tests in four L1–L2 communities: Russian-Hebrew, English-Hebrew, Russian-German, and Turkish-English. We compare the children's performance with monolingual norms, and consider effects of age of onset (AoO) and length of exposure (LoE) on performance.

Russian-Hebrew and English-Hebrew: A Study of Sentence Repetition in Sequential Bilingual Preschool Children Using Sentence Repetition with Pictures from the Goralnik Diagnostic Test of Hebrew

This section illustrates how a sample of sequential bilingual preschool children performed in the sentence repetition subtest of the *Goralnik Screening Test for Hebrew* (Goralnik, 1995), which is widely used in clinical settings in Israel for distinguishing between children with and without SLI . The Goralnik sentence repetition subtest has been normed for monolingual Hebrew-speaking children aged 3 to 6 years from high and low SES backgrounds, and provides norms for each SES group as well as combined norms. But do these norms hold for sequential bilingual children? And how is L2 children's performance on this sentence repetition task affected by AoO and LoE?

Description of the sentence repetition task

The Goralnik sentence repetition subtest consists of five complex sentences, each describing a different picture, so that sentence repetition is presented in a pictorial context. The experimental sentences vary in length and complexity. In terms of length, the sentences range from 4 to 7 words, and from 7 to 11 morphemes, excluding verb inflections. Examples (1) and (2) illustrate the shortest (4 words, 7 morphemes) and longest (6 words, 11 morphemes) sentences as measured in morphemes:

(1) *ha-yeled   mitnadned ve-ha-yalda   oxelet*
     The-boy swings   and-the-girl eats
     'The boy swings and the girl eats'.
(2) *ha-yeled paxad she-ha-balon   yauf   lo   me-ha-yad*
     The-boy feared that-the-ballon will-fly to-him of-the-hand
     'The boy was afraid that the balloon would fly out of his hand'.

In terms of clausal complexity, all five sentences have two clauses and vary in the types of complexity, including coordination, finite and non-finite sentential complements, relative clauses, and direct speech, with one sentence for each structure. In terms of content, all sentences make use of basic vocabulary for topics familiar to preschool children, e.g. everyday events/actions involving people, animals, toys, and vehicles, as illustrated by the above examples.

Methodology

Participants

Seventy-five TD sequential bilingual Russian-Hebrew children (40 female) and 35 TD sequential bilingual English-Hebrew children (20 female) participated in the study. The Russian-Hebrew children had a mean age of 5;10 (range: 4;10–6;11, SD: 6 months), and the English-Hebrew children a mean age of 5;9 (range: 4;5–6;6; SD: 6 months).

All children came from the same (mid-to-high) SES background, as defined by the mother's educational level. Both groups of L2 children were from L1 communities in the central part of Israel and attended preschools with no more than 50% children speaking their L1. They were growing up in families in which the language spoken at home was either Russian or English, and children did not have any history of speech and/or language delay or impairment, based on parental and school report.

Information about the L2 children's Age of Onset (AoO), Length of Exposure (LoE), and quantity and quality of input was collected through a parental and child questionnaire. AoO and LoE data for the two samples are presented in Table 3.1.

Procedure

The children participated in a battery of standardized and non-standardized assessments and experimental tasks. Testing was carried out in a quiet

Table 3.1 Age of onset (AoO) and length of exposure (LoE) in the Russian-Hebrew and English-Hebrew samples

	AoO in months	Breakdown of sample according to AoO in years			LoE in months	Breakdown of sample according to LoE in years		
	Mean (SD) Range	<2;0	2;0–3;0	>3;0	Mean (SD) Range	1–2	3–4	>4
Russian-Hebrew (*n* = 75)	35 (18) 0–66	22	24	29	37 (18) 12–75	23	34	18
English-Hebrew (*n* = 35)	35 (13) 6–51	7	6	22	34 (16) 15–69	14	16	5

room in the preschool. The sentences of the sentence repetition subtest from the Goralnik test were presented to the children by a native speaker of Hebrew. Children were told that they had to repeat each sentence verbatim. The children's responses were audio-recorded and were also scored manually on an answer sheet during the session.

Scoring

The children's responses were scored using the guidelines from the Goralnik manual, which awards a score of 6, 3 or 0 for each response. A score of 6 is given for a verbatim repetition (e.g. *ha-yeled axal tapuax ve-ha-yalda kar'a sefer* 'The boy ate an apple and the girl read a book'), a score of 3 for repetition of all major components with minor deviations (e.g. *ha-yeled axal tapuax ve-hi kar'a sefer* 'The boy ate an apple and she read a book'), and a score of 0 for a repetition that lacks some of the major constructs, such as subject, verb, or object, that appear in the original sentence (e.g. *ha-yeled axal ve-ha-yalda kar'a sefer* 'The boy ate and the girl read a book'). The final score is the sum of the scores on all items (maximum = 30). The Goralnik provides monolingual norms for raw scores. The z-scores were calculated based on the monolingual norms. The z-scores reflect the distance from the mean score in SDs.

Results

Table 3.2 shows the mean z-scores, standard deviations and ranges for the Russian-Hebrew and English-Hebrew children on the sentence repetition task. The mean scores for both groups were within the monolingual normal range.

Table 3.2 Results on Goralnik sentence repetition for Russian-Hebrew and English-Hebrew groups

	Russian-Hebrew (n = 75)			English-Hebrew (n = 35)		
	Mean	SD	Range	Mean	SD	Range
z-score	0.11	(0.89)	−2.36 to 1.05	0.31	(0.75)	−1.69 to 1.28

Table 3.3 Number of children scoring above, within and below normal range

	Russian-Hebrew (n = 75)	English-Hebrew (n = 35)
1 or more SD above	10 (13%)	4 (11%)
Within normal range	56 (75%)	28 (80%)
1 to 2 SD below	6 (8%)	3 (9%)
2 SD or more below	3 (4%)	0 (0%)

Breakdown of Russian-Hebrew and English-Hebrew sentence repetition performance according to monolingual norms

To investigate how children performed in terms of monolingual norms, we calculated the number of children who scored above the monolingual normal range (above 1 SD), within the monolingual normal range (below 1 SD and above −1 SD), between 1 and 2 SDs below the mean, and at or below −2 SD. Results are illustrated in Table 3.3.

Most of the bilingual children performed within the normal range; only 12 children in the combined sample performed below −1 SD, of whom only three children scored below −2 SDs. The profile of performance in these groups was therefore largely in line with norms and in fact slightly skewed towards the upper end (which might reflect the nature of the sample, with both groups from mid-to-high SES backgrounds and excluding children with any history of difficulties).

Analysis of performance by AoO

To investigate effects of AoO, we split the groups of L2 children into one group with AoO between 0;0 and 2;0, a second group with AoO between 2;1 and 3;0, and a third group with AoO between 3;1 and 5;4, as shown in Table 3.4.

For the Russian-Hebrew bilinguals, a one-way ANOVA showed a significant difference ($F (2, 72) = 4.212$, $p = 0.019$) traced by a post hoc Tukey test to a significant difference between the group with the lowest AoO and that with the highest AoO ($p = 0.013$). Similarly, for the English-Hebrew bilinguals, a one-way ANOVA showed a significant difference ($F (2, 32) = 3.413$, $p = 0.045$), traced by a post hoc Tukey test to a significant difference between the group with the lowest AoO and that with the highest AoO ($p = 0.039$).

Table 3.4 Breakdown of sentence repetition performance by AoO

	AoO 0;0 to 2;0				AoO 2;1 to 3;0				AoO 3;1 to 5;4			
	N	Mean	SD	Range	N	Mean	SD	Range	N	Mean	SD	Range
Russian-Hebrew	22	0.51	(0.43)	−0.16 to 1.05	24	0.11	(0.79)	−1.75 to 1.05	29	−0.19	(1.11)	−2.36 to 1.05
English-Hebrew	7	0.88	(0.21)	0.39 to 1.01	6	0.44	(0.48)	−1.6 to 0.94	22	0.14	(0.82)	−1.69 to 1.28

Table 3.5 Number of children scoring above, within and below normal range according to AoO

	AoO 0;0 to 2;0 (n = 29)	AoO 2;1 to 3;0 (n = 30)	AoO 3;1 to 5;4 (n = 51)
1 or more SD above	6 (21%)	1 (3%)	7 (13%)
Within normal range	23 (79%)	26 (87%)	35 (69%)
1 to 2 SD below	0 (0%)	3 (10%)	6 (12%)
2 SD or more below	0 (0%)	0 (0%)	3 (6%)

To investigate effects of AoO on how children performed in terms of monolingual norms, we merged the two samples and then calculated the number of children who scored above the monolingual normal range (above 1 SD), within the monolingual normal range (below 1SD and above −1 SD), between 1 and 2 SDs below the mean, and at or below −2 SD within each AoO range (see Table 3.5).

All children with AoO of 2;0 and below performed within or above the monolingual normal range. Of the 30 children with AoO of 2;1 to 3;0, only 3 (10%) performed below the monolingual normal range; however, of the 51 children with AoO of 3;1 to 5;4, 9 (17.65%) performed below the monolingual normal range. Notably, all of those who performed at least 2 SD below the mean were in the latest AoO group.

Analysis of performance by LoE

To investigate effects of LoE, we split the groups of L2 children into three groups with 1 to 2 years of exposure, 2;1 to 4 years of exposure and 4;1 to 6 years of exposure, as shown in Table 3.6.

All children with more than 4 years of exposure were within or above the monolingual normal range, and the three children who performed more than 2 SD below the monolingual mean had less than 4 years of exposure. For the Russian-Hebrew bilinguals, a one-way ANOVA showed no significant difference between the performance of L2 children in the different exposure groups ($F_{(2,72)} = 2.137$, $p = 0.125$). For the English-Hebrew bilinguals, a one-way

Table 3.6 Breakdown of sentence repetition performance by LoE

	LoE 1 to 2 years				LoE 2;1 to 4 years				LoE 4;1 to 6 years			
	N	Mean	SD	Range	N	Mean	SD	Range	N	Mean	SD	Range
Russian-Hebrew	23	−0.08	(1.07)	−2.36 to 1.05	34	0.04	(0.90)	−2.36 to 1.05	18	0.47	(0.48)	−0.16 to 1.05
English-Hebrew	14	−0.10	(0.79)	−1.69 to 1.28	16	0.52	(0.64)	−1.25 to 1.01	5	0.83	0.24	0.39 to 0.94

ANOVA showed a significant difference between the performance of L2 children (F (2,32) = 4.878, p = 0.014), traced by a post hoc Tukey test to a significant difference between the shortest exposure group and the longest exposure group (p = 0.032), and between the shortest exposure group and the medium exposure group (p = 0.043), with no significant difference between the medium and longest exposure groups.

Summary of Russian-Hebrew and English-Hebrew Findings

The findings in the L2 Hebrew studies (with L1 Russian or English) show that the majority of children (88% and 91% respectively) perform within or above the normal range for monolingual children despite variations in exposure. Only three out of a combined group of 110 children, all three of whom were exposed to Hebrew after the age of three, fell more than 2 SDs below the monolingual mean. The overall distribution of performance of this bilingual group in the L2 is therefore in line with the normal monolingual distribution, making sentence repetition a promising tool for use in L2 assessment of this population. Nevertheless, results indicate that age of onset and length of exposure need to be taken into account, and some caution exercised in interpreting low scores when a child's exposure to the language has been limited.

Russian-German: A Study of Sentence Repetition in Sequential Bilingual Preschool Children using the Sprachstandscreening für das Vorschulalter (Grimm, 2003) for German

This section illustrates how a sample of sequential bilingual preschool children performed on the Sprachstandscreening für das Vorschulalter (Grimm, 2003), a sentence repetition task that is used in clinical settings in

Germany (Berlin) for distinguishing between children with and without SLI. The sentence repetition task has been normed for monolingual children from high and low SES backgrounds. Again, the question is whether these norms hold for sequential bilingual children, and how the L2 children's performance on this sentence repetition task is affected by the AoO and LoE.

Description of the sentence repetition task

The Sprachstandscreening für das Vorschulalter consists of 15 sentences, six semantically sensible sentences and nine semantically anomalous sentences, which vary in length and complexity. In terms of length, the sentences range from 6 to 10 words. Examples (3) and (4) illustrate the shortest and longest sentences as measured in words:

(3)   *Die Ente sitzt neben   dem Auto*
      The duck sits beside the car
      'The duck is sitting beside the car'.
(4)   *Der Schmutzige Hund wird vom   Vater in der Wanne   gebadet*
      The dirty   dog   is   by the father in the bathtub bathed
      'The dirty dog is being bathed by the father in the bathtub'.

In terms of sentence complexity, of the six semantically sensible sentences, four sentences comprise simple clauses (two in the passive voice, as exemplified by (4) above), and two have adverbial modifiers (one of which is a whole clause):

(5)   *Vor   dem Schlafen putzen Kinder   die Zähne*
      Before the sleep   brush children the teeth
      'Before sleeping the children brush their teeth'
(6)   *Die Kinder   lachen, weil   sie   auf dem Bett hüpfen*
      The children laugh because they on the bed jump
      'The children are laughing because they are jumping on the bed'.

Of the semantically anomalous sentences, five sentences comprise simple clauses (two in the passive voice), e.g. (7), and four sentences have two clauses, two with a relative clause and two with adverbials, e.g. (8):

(7)   *Der Kindergarten   wird von den roten Bären geschüttelt*
      The Kindergarten is   by the red   bears shaken
      'The Kindergarten is shaken by the red bears'
(8)   *Bevor   der Goldfisch hinfällt, frisst er aus dem Fenster*
      Before the goldfish falls,   eats it off the window
      'Before the goldfish falls down, it eats from the window'.

In terms of content, all sentences make use of basic vocabulary for topics familiar to preschool children, e.g. everyday events/actions involving people, animals, furniture, vehicles, as illustrated in the above examples. Unlike the Hebrew standardized test, the sentences in the German standardized test are presented without pictures.

Methodology

Participants

Sixty-one typically developing (TD) sequential bilingual Russian-German children (30 female) participated in the study. These children had a mean age of 5;6 (range: 3;11–7;2, SD: 10 months). In terms of SES, calculated by parents' education, 25 out of the 61 fathers and 32 out of 61 mothers had less than 12 years of education (i.e. high school), whereas the other parents had more than 13 years of education (i.e. high school and some further education). This yielded two SES groups, high and low, as measured by mothers' educations.

The Russian-German children were from the Russian community in Berlin, Germany, and attended preschools with no more than 50% Russian-speaking children. They were growing up in families in which the language spoken at home was Russian, and had no history of speech and/or language delay or impairment based on parental and school report.

Information about the L2 children's Age of Onset (AoO), Length of Exposure (LoE), quantity and quality of input was collected through a parental and child questionnaire. AoO and LoE data for this sample are presented in Table 3.7.

Procedure

The children participated in a battery of standardized and non-standardized assessments and experimental tasks. Testing was carried out in a quiet

Table 3.7 Age of onset (AoO) and length of exposure (LoE) in the Russian-German sample

	AoO in months	Breakdown of sample according to AoO in years			LoE in months	Breakdown of sample according to LoE in years		
	Mean (SD) Range	<2;0	2;0 to 3;0	>3;0	Mean (SD) Range	1 to 2	3 to 4	>4
Russian-German (n = 61)	24 (10) 0–46	37	14	10	42 (15) 13–82	7	31	23

room in the preschool. The sentences of the German sentence repetition task were presented to the children by a native speaker of German, and children were told that they had to repeat each sentence verbatim. The children's responses were audio-recorded and were also marked manually on an answer sheet during the session.

Scoring

The children's responses were scored using the guidelines from the Sprachstandscreening für das Vorschulalter (Grimm, 2003) manual.

To calculate raw scores, the number of words repeated correctly was counted. The z-scores were calculated based on the monolingual norms. The z-scores reflect the distance from the mean monolingual score in SDs.

Results

Comparison between low SES and high SES Russian-German children

Table 3.8 shows the mean z-score, standard deviation and range for the Russian-German children on the sentence repetition task according to SES as measured by mothers' education.

A one-way ANOVA showed a near-significant difference between the two SES groups (F (1, 59) = 3.445, p = 0.068). This becomes significant if the cut-off point is 14 years of education rather than 12 years (F (1,59) = 4.667, p = 0.035). Nevertheless, the mean score for both groups was within the monolingual normal range.

Breakdown of Russian-German sentence repetition performance by SES according to monolingual norms

To investigate how children performed relative to monolingual norms, we calculated the number of children who scored above the monolingual normal range (above 1 SD), within the monolingual normal range (below 1 SD and above −1 SD), between 1 and 2 SDs below the mean, and at or below −2 SD. Results are illustrated in Table 3.9.

Two-thirds of the bilingual children performed within or above the monolingual normal range. Whereas a third of the sample performed below −1 SD, only three children's performance was more than 2 SDs below

Table 3.8 Results on German sentence repetition test according to SES

	Lower SES (n = 32)			Higher SES (n = 29)		
	Mean	SD	Range	Mean	SD	Range
z-score	−0.76	(0.66)	−2.20 to 0.4	−0.36	(1.02)	−2.90 to 1.60

Table 3.9 Number of children scoring above, within and below normal range

	Lower SES (n = 32)	Higher SES (n = 29)	Total (n = 61)
1 SD above	0 (0%)	3 (10%)	3 (5%)
Within norms	19 (59%)	21 (73%)	40 (66%)
1 to 2 SD below	12 (37%)	3 (10%)	15 (24%)
2 SD or more below	1 (4%)	2 (7%)	3 (5%)

the mean. Notably, though, in the lower SES group only 56% of the children performed within the monolingual normal range, compared with 76% of the children in the higher SES group.

Analysis of performance by AoO

To investigate effects of AoO, we split the group of L2 children into one group with AoO between 0;0 and 2;0 ($n = 37$), a second group with AoO between 2;1 and 3;0 ($n = 14$), and a third group with AoO between 3;1 and 3;10 ($n = 10$) as shown in Table 3.10.

For the Russian-German bilinguals, a one-way ANOVA showed no significant difference for AoO ($F (2, 58) = 0.241$, $p = 0.78$). Introducing the mother's education as a covariate had no impact on the results.

To investigate effects of AoO on how children performed in terms of monolingual norms, we calculated the number of children who scored above the monolingual normal range (above 1 SD), within the monolingual normal range (below 1SD and above –1 SD), between 1 and 2 SDs below the mean, and at or below –2 SD within each AoO range (see Table 3.11).

Three of the children with AoO of 2;0 or below performed above the monolingual normal range, and all the others were either within the monolingual normal range or no more than 1.7 SD below the mean. Of the 14 children with AoO of 2;1 to 3;0, 5 performed below the monolingual normal range, and of the 10 children with AoO of 3;1 to 3;10, 3 performed below the monolingual normal range. Notably, all of those who performed 2 SD below the mean were in the highest AoO groups.

Table 3.10 Breakdown of sentence repetition by AoO

AoO 0;0 to 2;0 (n = 37)			AoO 2;1 to 3;0 (n = 14)			AoO 3;1 to 3;10 (n = 10)		
Mean	SD	Range	Mean	SD	Range	Mean	SD	Range
–0.51	(0.81)	–1.70 to 1.60	–0.68	(0.96)	–2.90 to 0.90	–0.65	(1.01)	–2.30 to 0.40

Table 3.11 Number of children scoring above, within and below normal range according to AoO

	AoO 0;0 to 2;0 (n = 37)	AoO 2;1 to 3;0 (n = 14)	AoO 3;1 to 3;10 (n = 10)
1 SD above	3 (8%)	0 (0%)	0 (0%)
Within norms	24 (65%)	9 (64%)	7 (70%)
1 to 2 SD below	10 (27%)	4 (29%)	1 (10%)
2 SD or more below	0 (0%)	1 (7%)	2 (20%)

Analysis of performance by LoE

To investigate effects of LoE, we split the groups of L2 children into three groups with 1 to 2 years of exposure, 2;1 to 4 years of exposure, and 4;1 to 5;9 years of exposure, as shown in Table 3.12.

Most of the children with more than 4 years of exposure (87%) were within or above the monolingual normal range, and the three children who performed more than 2SD below the monolingual mean had less than 4 years of exposure, two of them with less than 2 years of exposure. A one-way ANOVA showed no significant difference, however, for LoE (F (2,58) = 2.243, p = 0.115). Introducing the mother's education as a covariate yields a near-significant difference (F (3,57) = 2.434, p = 0.074).

Summary of Russian-German Findings

The findings in the L2 German studies (with L1 Russian) show that over-all two-thirds of the bilingual children performed within or above the mono-lingual normal range, whereas 5% scored more than 2 SD below the mean. This distribution is notably lower than the normal monolingual distribution (especially considering the sample excluded children with language diffi-culties). The distribution in the higher SES group came closer to matching the normal monolingual distribution and included three children scoring above the normal range, but even so, higher than expected numbers fell below -2 SD (7%, compared with expected 2.3% in the normal monolingual

Table 3.12 Breakdown of sentence repetition by LoE

LoE 1;0 to 2;0 years (n = 7)			LoE 2;1 to 4;0 years (n = 31)			LoE 4;1 to 5;9 years (n = 23)		
Mean	SD	Range	Mean	SD	Range	Mean	SD	Range
−1.01	(0.77)	−2.30 to 0.10	−0.66	(0.92)	−2.90 to 1.60	−0.31	(0.76)	−1.70 to 1.20

distribution). Those scoring below –2 SD were exposed to German after the age of 2 and for less than 4 years. These outcomes demonstrate the need for some caution in using monolingual norms with this population, and the possible influence of SES, as well as language exposure, on children's performance.

Turkish-English: A Study of Sentence Repetition in Sequential Bilingual Children Using the Sentence Recall Subtest from CELF-3

This section illustrates how a sample of sequential Turkish-English bilingual children performed in the Sentence Recall subtest of the Clinical Evaluation of Language Fundamentals III (CELF-3) (Semel *et al.*, 2000). The CELF is widely used in clinical settings in the UK, and the Sentence Recall subtest has been shown to have a high degree of specificity and sensitivity in distinguishing between children with and without SLI (Conti-Ramsden *et al.*, 2001). However, it is unclear whether or not this will hold for sequential bilingual (L2) children. In order to address this question, we need to establish whether typically developing L2 children score within monolingual norms, and how their performance relates to their age of onset (AoO) and length of exposure (LoE). The following study compared the performance of typically developing Turkish-English children on CELF Sentence Recall relative to monolingual children, and investigated the effects of AoO and LoE.

Description of CELF Sentence Recall

The CELF Sentence Recall subtest consists of two practice and 26 test sentences. The test sentences vary in length, complexity, and content. In terms of length, the sentences range from 6 to 19 words. Examples (9) and (10) illustrate the shortest and longest sentence:

(9)   Did the girl catch the netball?
(10) The boy [who didn't turn up for practice] wasn't allowed to play for the team until a week later.

In terms of clausal complexity, sentences range from one to five clauses. (9) exemplifies a sentence with one clause, whereas examples (10)–(13) illustrate complex sentences. Sentence (10) includes a subject relative clause, (11) involves sentence coordination, (12) a truncated passive structure in embedded and main clauses, and (13) five clauses including one double embedding:

(11) [The fielder caught the ball] and [the crowd cheered loudly]

(12) [Before the first years were dismissed for lunch] [they were told to hand in their assignments].
(13) [When the students had finished studying] [they decided [to get something [to eat]] [before going home]].

In terms of pragmatic and lexical content, 16 out of the 26 sentences had a school-related topic involving school-related vocabulary (as illustrated by the above examples), and the remaining sentences were on other topics, e.g. games, everyday events involving people, and events involving animals and vehicles.

It is important to note that the factors of length, complexity, and topic are confounded in this task. The first six sentences on the test are relatively short, consist of one clause and most involve events that are not school-based. All other sentences are long, consist of multiple clauses, and their content almost always relates to activities around school. If children are successful in repeating the first six sentences and make errors in the remaining sentences, it is impossible to know whether they fail because of the length of the sentences, their complexity, or a lack of familiarity with the school-related vocabulary.

Methodology

Participants

Seventeen TD sequential bilingual Turkish-English children (8 female) and 15 TD age-matched monolingual English-speaking children (10 female) participated in the study. The L2 children had a mean age of 7;10 (range: 6;1–9;3; SD: 13 months), and the L1 children a mean age of 7;10 (range: 7;2–8;11; SD: 5 months) ($F (1, 30) = 0.36, p = 0.851$). Both groups of children attended schools whose percentage of free school meals was well above the national average, indicating low socioeconomic status. The L2 children were from the Turkish community in London, were growing up in families in which the language spoken at home was Turkish, and attended schools with a high density of Turkish-speaking children. The monolingual children were attending schools in Reading. Both samples excluded children with a history of speech and/or language delay or impairment based on parental and school report.

Information about the L2 children's age of onset (AoO), length of exposure (LoE), and quantity and quality of input was collected through a parental and child questionnaire. AoO and LoE data are presented in Table 3.13.

Procedure

The children participated in a battery of standardized and non-standardized assessments and experimental tasks. The Sentence Recall task from CELF-3 was recorded in the Speech Booth, a purpose-built sound-proof

Table 3.13 Age of onset (AoO) and length of exposure (LoE) in the Turkish-English sample (*n* = 17)

AoO in months	Breakdown of sample according to AoO in years		LoE in months	Breakdown of sample according to LoE in years	
Mean (SD)Range	<3;0	3;0–5;0	Mean (SD) Range	1–3	4–6
39	9	8	55	5	12
(6.6)			(17)		
29–60			21–83		

room, at the Department of Clinical Language Sciences, University of Reading. The sentences were digitally recorded at normal speed by a female speaker and merged into a single file using Adobe Audition.

A laptop was used for the presentation of this task. Sentences were presented to the children through headphones, and a microphone connected to the laptop was used to record the children's responses. This task does not include pictures. The children were told that they had to repeat each sentence verbatim. Their responses were recorded using Adobe Audition.

Scoring

The children's responses were scored as specified in the CELF manual. To calculate raw scores, each sentence is given a score of 3 if it is repeated verbatim, a score of 2 if there is one error, a score of 1 if there are two or three errors, and a score of 0 if there are four or more errors. Standard scores were calculated based on the monolingual norms from CELF (mean = 10, SD = 3). The z-scores were calculated from the standard scores.

Results

Comparison between L2 and L1 children

Table 3.14 reports the standard and z-scores of the L2 and L1 children on the Sentence Recall task.

Although the mean for the L1 group fell just short of the population mean, the L2 group mean was almost two standard deviations below. A one-way ANOVA using the standard scores confirmed that the L2 children were significantly less accurate than the L1 children (F (1, 31) = 45.29, $p < 0.001$).

Breakdown of L1 and L2 Sentence Recall performance according to monolingual norms

To compare the distribution of performance in each group with the monolingual normal distribution, we calculated the number of children that

Table 3.14 Results on CELF Sentence Recall for L1 and L2 groups

| | L1 (n = 15) | | | L2 (n = 17) | | |
	Mean	SD	Range	Mean	SD	Range
Standard score	9.5	(2.3)	5–13	4.5	(2.1)	3–10
z-score	−0.2	(0.8)	−1.7 to 1	−1.8	(0.7)	−2.3 to 0

Table 3.15 Number of children scoring above, within and below normal range

	L1 (n = 15)	L2 (n = 17)
1 SD above	0	0
Within norms	13 (87%)	2 (12%)
1 to 2 SD below	2 (13%)	3 (18%)
2 SD or more below	0 (0%)	12 (70%)

scored above the monolingual normal range (above 1 SD), within the monolingual normal range (below 1 SD and above −1 SD), between 1 and 2 SDs below the mean, and at or below −2 SD. Results are illustrated in Table 3.15.

It is notable that no child in these samples scored above the monolingual normal range. However, most of the monolingual children (87%) performed within the L1 normal range, with only two children (13%) performing between 1 and 2 SDs below the L1 mean, and no child scoring below −2 SD. The exact opposite pattern was observed in the group of L2 children. Only two children (12%) performed within the L1 normal range, while three children (18%) performed between 1 and 2 SDs below the L1 mean, and the majority (70%) performed below −2 SDs.

Analysis of L2 performance by AoO and LoE

To investigate whether or not AoO affected the L2 children's performance, we divided the group of L2 children into groups with AoO between 2;5 and 3;0 years (n = 9) and between 3;3 and 5 years (n = 8). Results are shown in Table 3.16.

Table 3.16 Breakdown of L2 Sentence Recall performance according to AoO

| | AoO 2;5 to 3;0 (n = 9) | | | AoO 3;3 to 5;0 (n = 8) | | |
	Mean	SD	Range	Mean	SD	Range
Standard score	5	(2.5)	3–10	4	(1.3)	3–7
z-score	−1.7	(0.8)	−2.3 to 0	−2	(0.4)	−2.3 to −1

Table 3.17 Breakdown of L2 Sentence Recall performance according to LoE

	LoE 1 to 3 years (n = 5)			LoE 4 to 6 years (n = 12)		
	Mean	SD	Range	Mean	SD	Range
Standard score	4	(0)	4	4.8	(2.5)	3–10
z-score	−2	(0)	−2	−1.7	(0.8)	−2.3 to 0

A one-way ANOVA using the standard scores showed no significant difference between the performance of L2 children with lower vs higher AoO (F (1,16) = 1.54, p = 0.233).

To investigate whether LoE affected the L2 children's accuracy, we divided the children into a group with 1 to 3 years of exposure (n = 5) and a group with 4 to 6 years of exposure (n = 12). Results are shown in Table 3.17.

A one-way ANOVA using the standard scores showed no significant difference between the performance of L2 children with shorter vs longer exposure (F (1,16) = 0.69, p = 0.421).

Analysis by sentence type

As pointed out above, the sentences in the CELF Sentence Recall task become progressively longer and more complex. Given the sensitivity of sentence repetition to morphosyntactic knowledge in simple sentences (see above), it is useful to investigate how length/complexity affected performance in the L1 and L2 groups. Table 3.18 shows the raw scores for the short/simple sentences (1–6) vs the long/complex sentences (7–26) in the two groups (maximum score for short sentences: 18; maximum score for long sentences: 60) and corresponding percentage correct.

To compare the groups on the two sentence types, we conducted a mixed ANOVA on the percentage correct with Group (L2 vs L1) as a

Table 3.18 Mean raw scores and percentages on short/simple vs long/complex sentences according to group

		L1 (n = 15)			L2 (n = 17)		
		Mean	SD	Range	Mean	SD	Range
Short/simple	Raw	17.5	(1.3)	13–18	14.6	(3.2)	9–18
sentences	%	97%	(7.2)	72–100%	81.4%	(17.6)	50–100%
(max = 18)							
Long/complex	Raw	18.1	(7.7)	6–33	4.2	(6.5)	0–21
sentences	%	30.2%	(12.8)	10–55%	7.1%	(10.8)	0–35%
(max = 60)							

between-subjects factor and Sentence Type (short/simple vs long/complex) as a within-subjects factor. This showed a main effect of Group (F (1,30) = 24.07, $p<0.001$), reflecting lower accuracy of the L2 children, and a main effect of Sentence Type (F (1,30) = 1021.26, $p<0.001$), reflecting lower accuracy on complex compared to simple sentences. There was no significant interaction between Group and Sentence Type, which shows that both groups had lower accuracy on complex than on simple sentences.

Summary of Turkish-English Findings

This study included Turkish-English sequential bilingual children and monolingual children attending schools of similar SES, as judged by the criterion of above-average percentage of free school meals. The results showed that the distribution of the monolingual children on the sentence recall task from CELF was in line with monolingual norms. However, the sequential bilingual children were less accurate than the monolingual children, and a striking 70% of the L2 children performed at least 2SD below the monolingual mean. The AoO in the L2 group, ranging from 2;5 to 5;0 years, and length of exposure, ranging from 1 to 6 years, were not found to affect performance. In considering these findings, it is important to note that none of the children were exposed to English before the age of 2;5, and they were attending schools with a high density of children speaking Turkish. Finally, sentence length and complexity affected both L1 and L2 children in a similar way. Both groups performed better on short and simple sentences than on long and complex sentences. The results of this study highlight the need for caution in interpreting results on the CELF sentence recall task in this population.

Discussion

The results of these studies of sentence repetition in L2 are strikingly divergent. The findings in the L2 Hebrew studies (with L1 Russian/English) are promising for use of sentence repetition in L2 assessment, with the majority of children (88% and 91%) performing in the normal range for monolingual children despite variations in exposure, and only three out of a combined group of 110 children falling more than 2 SDs below the monolingual mean. The overall distribution of performance is in line with the normal monolingual distribution. Based on these findings, any child scoring outside the normal monolingual range may be considered at risk of language impairment. However, this is not the case for the L1 Turkish/L2 English study, where the majority of L2 children (70%) scored more than 2 SDs below the monolingual mean, and only 2 of the 17 children obtained scores in the normal monolingual range. Thus, if monolingual norms were applied, the majority of these children would be identified as impaired. The Russian-German group fell between these extremes, with 66% scoring within or above the normal monolingual range, but a notable 29% between 1 and 2 SDs below the mean, and 5% even lower.

Sources of difference

The three studies we have reported vary in multiple respects apart from language pairs and countries of residence of participants. This multiplicity of differences between studies precludes direct comparison of findings. However, analyses *within* studies indicate factors that may influence sentence repetition performance, and these throw some light on likely sources of divergence between studies. Consideration of these factors is important for drawing interim conclusions about the use of sentence repetition and for identifying further research needed to clarify the contribution of sentence repetition to assessment in L2 populations.

Age of onset and length of exposure

The age range, AoO, and LoE of participants varied between and within studies, as summarised in Table 3.19.

The Hebrew study found effects of AoO and a trend towards effects of LoE. It is perhaps unsurprising that children exposed between 0 and 2;0 years, who might be considered simultaneous bilinguals, perform like monolingual children. But results were good even for those exposed after age 3;0, with 82% performing in the normal range, including 13% who were more than 1 SD above the monolingual mean. In the Russian-German study, AoO and LoE did not prove significant factors (although the children scoring below −2 SD had the latest AoO and shortest LoE, and exploratory correlational analyses, not shown above, suggested a significant correlation of performance with LoE, $r(60) = 0.279$, $p = 0.03$). These factors also proved non-significant in the Turkish-English study. Although the relatively small numbers in that study reduced power to identify effects, AoO and LoE within the sample varied widely, so the lack of effects is striking. As no child in the Turkish-English study was exposed before 2;5 years, it is possible that

Table 3.19 Mean (range) for age, age of onset, length of exposure in the four L2 groups (all given in months)

Study	Age	AoO	LoE
Russian-Hebrew (*n* = 75)	70 (58–83)	35 (0–66)	37 (12–75)
English-Hebrew (*n* = 35)	69 (53–78)	35 (6–51)	34 (15–69)
Russian-German (*n* = 61)	66 (47–86)	24 (0–46)	42 (13–82)
Turkish-English (n = 17)	106 (73–111)	39 (29–60)	55 (21–83)

this is a turning-point for age of onset, but our findings suggest other factors are at stake. Indices of AoO and LoE used in these studies provide a limited measure of children's language experience: following first exposure, the balance of language use at home and at school might vary widely. It is notable that the L2 children in the Turkish-English study were attending schools with a high density of Turkish-speaking children. Teasing out the effects of more subtle differences in language experience would require more detailed information about exposure and careful control of this factor.

Our studies highlight another potentially important factor which may be related to differences in language exposure, namely SES.

SES

The SES of participant groups varied between our studies. The Russian-German study included two SES groups, allowing within-study comparison of SES effects. This revealed significant differences by SES, as measured according to mothers' level of education (more vs less than 14 years of education). It is possible that SES differences overlapped with differences in AoO and LoE, but as AoO and LoE were not significant in this study, we have some indication that SES was influential. SES might also be implicated in the very poor sentence repetition performance observed in the Turkish-English group. Although information about the SES levels of the individuals in this group was limited, all were attending schools in the low SES category according to the 'free school meals' index. In contrast, the high performing children in the Hebrew study were all from mid-to-high SES backgrounds.

SES is by no means a simple factor (Roy & Chiat, 2013), and whatever indices of SES are used, they may be compounded with cultural differences. Nonetheless, the suggestion that SES may be an important factor in sentence repetition performance of L2 children is in line with findings of SES effects in monolingual children (see introductory section of this chapter).

Test materials

The sentence repetition tests administered to the children differed in content and scoring. Sentence presentation is accompanied by pictures in the Hebrew test, but not in the German and English tests. The German test includes plausible and implausible sentences, whereas the Hebrew and English tests include only plausible targets. Sentences in the Hebrew and German tests are made up of early-acquired vocabulary, and although they contain complex structures, sentence complexity is limited. In contrast, the CELF sentence recall subtest administered to the Turkish-English group is designed for school-age children (up to age 21), and after the first six single-clause sentences, targets become progressively more complex. Almost all sentences deploy later-acquired and often school-related vocabulary. Scoring in the Hebrew and English tests is based on types and numbers of errors per sentence, respectively, whereas the German test scores number of words correct.

The substantially greater linguistic demands of the CELF sentence recall task could be responsible for the particularly poor performance observed in the Turkish-English group. However, comparison of L2 with L1 performance on the simple and complex targets within this task did not reveal an interaction between complexity and group, indicating that the L2 group had difficulties with simple as well as complex targets.

Implications for L2 assessment

The heterogeneous levels of L2 performance within our three studies demonstrate that the tests are tapping into children's linguistic skills. This is as we would expect from studies of sentence repetition in typically and atypically developing monolingual children, and from Polišenská's evidence that linguistic knowledge, particularly morphosyntactic and lexical knowledge, affects children's repetition capacity. Sentence repetition is therefore a useful tool for assessing linguistic *proficiency* in L2 children. As such, it has all the advantages identified for sentence repetition as a language assessment for L1 (see introductory sections). With a limited number of carefully controlled stimuli, sentence repetition is quick to administer and score and reveals not only level of language proficiency but strengths and weaknesses in targeted aspects of language. Sentence repetition tasks therefore provide an efficient and informative method for checking levels of language in L2 groups and individuals. Testing children's sentence repetition may expose low levels of language performance that have been overlooked or confused with low ability. In so doing, it would highlight ways in which school language needs to be tailored to the L2 population in the school, and indicate language needs that require additional support at a group and/or individual level. Taking the example of the Turkish-English group reported in this chapter, it is important for teachers to know that these children's ability to process sentence input in English is at a level that would be deemed impaired in their monolingual peers and to consider the support needed to raise their language to an appropriate level and facilitate their access to the school curriculum.

In monolingual children, low proficiency is assumed to reflect low ability unless there is reason to think children's language environment has been unusually limited. In the case of L2 acquisition, we cannot assume that proficiency reflects ability as experience is known to vary. Individually and collectively, our studies provide extensive evidence that sentence repetition performance is heavily influenced by the heterogeneous experience of L2 children. In the Hebrew studies, AoO and LoE were found to have an effect, indicating the need to take these factors into account in judging performance. However, the Russian-German and Turkish-English studies revealed that sentence repetition may be more affected by differences in children's experience that go beyond age of onset and years of exposure and led to the suggestion that late onset and reduced exposure associated with L2 acquisition may be further compounded by limitations in language environment associated with low SES background. The disproportionate numbers of children in the Turkish-English and Russian-German studies performing in the range associated with impaired monolingual performance highlight the need for caution in using sentence repetition tests designed and normed for monolingual children for clinical assessment of L2 children.

Based on our findings, we conclude that monolingual norms on a sentence repetition task can be applied if assessing children's *proficiency* in L2. However, they cannot be applied for purposes of clinical diagnosis unless there is adequate evidence that children in the relevant L2 population with a similar level of exposure perform in line with these norms (as in the L2 Hebrew groups).

Future directions

Difficulties with morphosyntax, and specifically with function words and inflections, are a hallmark of SLI in English (Leonard, 1998), and are apparent in children's sentence repetition (Chiat & Roy, 2008; Seeff-Gabriel *et al.*, 2008, 2010). Although function word repetition was also found to be low in the socially disadvantaged group studied by Roy and Chiat, this was not the case for the oldest age group, in which the rate of low performance was in line with norms (Roy & Chiat, 2013). As discussed above, the extent of poor performance in the Turkish-English group might in part be attributable to the vocabulary and syntax sampled in the CELF sentence recall test. We suggest that a test targeting more basic vocabulary and morphosyntax, while less informative about language proficiency needed for school purposes, might be more effective in distinguishing L2 children with language deficits from those with limited proficiency.

As a next step in evaluating the potential of sentence repetition in L2 clinical assessment, we propose an investigation of performance on a repetition test comprising simple sentences that are made up of early-acquired vocabulary and include representative exemplars of the morphosyntactic devices used to convey relations in the target language (word order, function words, inflections). Administration of such a test to L2 groups varying in SES as well as AoO and LoE will reveal the effects of these factors on attainment of core sentence structure and the point at which the test is valid for identifying deficits that require clinical intervention. Systematically controlled stimuli allow qualitative as well as quantitative scoring of morphosyntactic targets. This will reveal whether L2 groups show particular profiles of omission or commission errors (see Armon-Lotem, 2010; Paradis, 2010), and whether a small proportion of children lag behind or produce different errors from their L2 peers. Ideally, L2 children would be assessed using analogous sentence repetition tests in L1, to evaluate consistency of performance across languages and to determine whether children deemed at risk in one language are also found to be at risk in the other.

A programme of research along the lines we have proposed is currently being pursued under the auspices of COST Action IS0804 (http://www.bi-sli.org/). The multi-country team of researchers involved in this Action have drawn up a framework for constructing a sentence repetition test that targets a comprehensive range of simple and complex sentence functions. Applied to particular languages, this framework can be 'filled in' and extended to ensure representative sampling of syntactic and morphosyntactic devices deployed by each language. Results of sentence repetition tests using this framework in a range of typologically varied language pairs will provide extensive evidence to address questions raised by the preliminary investigations that we have reported, including effects of children's exposure and experience in L1 and L2, linguistic characteristics of L1 and L2, and socioeconomic/sociocultural factors. Given the value of sentence repetition as a measure of language proficiency, and as a clinical language assessment in L1, the provision of well-founded sentence repetition tests with normative data for different samples of children will help with clinical assessment of sequential bilingual children and those from minority language backgrounds.

Acknowledgements

The data collection for the English-Hebrew study was funded by the Israel Science Foundation (Grant 938). The data collection for the Russian-Hebrew and Russian-German studies was supported by the BMBF funded Consortium 'Migration and Societal Integration', grant number 01UW0702B. The data collection for the Turkish-English study was supported by the Economic and Social Research Council grant number RES-061-23-0137. The writing of this paper was supported by COST Action IS0804 'Language Impairment in a Multilingual Society: Linguistic Patterns and the Road to Assessment'.

References

Archibald, L.M. and Gathercole, S.E. (2006) Nonword repetition: A comparison of tests. *Journal of Speech, Language, and Hearing Research* 49, 970–983.
Armon-Lotem, S. (2010) Instructive bilingualism: Can bilingual children with specific language impairment rely on one language in learning a second one? *Applied Psycholinguistics* 31, 253–260.
Bishop, D.V.M., McDonald, D., Bird, S. and Hayiou-Thomas, M.E. (2009) Children who read words accurately despite language impairment: Who are they and how do they do it? *Child Development* 80, 593–605.
Brown, R. (1973) *A First Language*. Harmondsworth: Penguin.
Campbell, T., Dollaghan, C., Needleman, H. and Janosky, J. (1997) Reducing bias in language assessment: Processing-dependent measures. *Journal of Speech, Language, and Hearing Research* 40, 519–525.

Casalini, C., Brizzolara, D., Chilosi, A., Cipriani, P., Marcolini, S., Pecini, C., Roncoli, S. and Burani, C. (2007) Nonword repetition in children with Specific Language Impairment: A deficit in phonological working memory or in long-term verbal knowledge? *Cortex* 43, 769–776.

Coady, J.A. and Evans, J.L. (2008) Uses and interpretations of non-word repetition tasks in children with and without language impairments (SLI). *International Journal of Language and Communication Disorders* 43, 1–40.

Conti-Ramsden, G., Botting, N. and Faragher, B. (2001) Psycholinguistic markers for specific language impairment (SLI). *Journal of Child Psychology and Psychiatry* 42, 741–748.

Devescovi, A. and Caselli, M.C. (2007) Sentence repetition as a measure of early grammatical development in Italian. *International Journal of Language and Communication Disorders* 42, 187–208.

Dollaghan, C. and Campbell, T.F. (1998) Nonword repetition and child language impairment. *Journal of Speech, Language, and Hearing Research* 41, 1136–1146.

Engel, P.M.J., Santos, F.H. and Gathercole, S.E. (2008) Are working memory measures free of socioeconomic influence? *Journal of Speech, Language, and Hearing Research* 51, 1580–1587.

Fraser, C., Bellugi, U. and Brown, R. (1963) Control of grammar in imitation, comprehension, and production. *Journal of Verbal Learning & Verbal Behavior* 2, 121–135.

Gathercole, S.E. (2006) Nonword repetition and word learning: The nature of the relationship. *Applied Psycholinguistics* 27, 513–543.

Gathercole, S.E. and Baddeley, A.D. (1989) Evaluation of the role of phonological STM in the development of vocabulary in children: A longitudinal study. *Journal of Memory and Language* 28, 200–213.

Gathercole, V.C.M. (2010) Interface or face to face? The profiles and contours of bilinguals and specific language impairment. *Applied Psycholinguistics* 31, 282–293.

Girbau, D. and Schwartz, R.G. (2007) Non-word repetition in Spanish-speaking children with Specific Language Impairment (SLI). *International Journal of Language and Communication Disorders* 42, 59–75.

Goralnik, E. (1995) *Goralnik Diagnostic Test*. Even Yehuda, Israel: Matan.

Graf Estes, K., Evans, J.L. and Else-Quest, N.M. (2007) Differences in the nonword repetition performance of children with and without Specific Language Impairment: A meta-analysis. *Journal of Speech, Language, and Hearing Research* 50, 177–195.

Grimm, H. (2003) Sprachstandsscreening für das Vorschulalter. Göttingen/Bern/Toronto/Seattle: Hogrefe.

Leonard, L.B. (1998) *Children with Specific Language Impairment*. Cambridge, MA: MIT Press.

Newcomer, P.L. and Hammill, D.D. (1997) *Test of Language Development. Primary* (3rd edn). (*TOLD-P:3*). Austin, Texas: Pro-Ed.

Paradis, J. (2010) The interface between bilingual development and specific language impairment. *Applied Psycholinguistics* 31, 227–252.

Polišenská, K. (2011) *The influence of linguistic structure on memory span: Repetition tasks as a measure of language ability*. PhD thesis, City University London.

Polišenská, K., Chiat, S. and Roy, P. (under review) The contribution of linguistic knowledge to immediate verbal recall in children.

Redmond, S.M. (2005) Differentiating SLI from ADHD using children's sentence recall and production of past tense morphology. *Clinical Linguistics and Phonetics* 19, 109–127.

Redmond, S.M., Thompson, H.L. and Goldstein, S. (2011) Psycholinguistic profiling differentiates Specific Language Impairment from typical development and from Attention-Deficit/Hyperactivity Disorder. *Journal of Speech, Language, and Hearing Research* 54, 99–117.

Riches, N.G., Loucas, T., Baird, G., Charman, T. and Simonoff, E. (2010) Sentence repetition in adolescents with specific language impairments and autism: An investigation of complex syntax. *International Journal of Language and Communication Disorders* 45, 47–60.

Roy, P. and Chiat, S. (2004) A prosodically controlled word and nonword repetition task for 2- to 4-year-olds: Evidence from typically developing children. *Journal of Speech, Language, and Hearing Research* 47, 223–34.

Roy, P. and Chiat, S. (2013) Teasing apart disadvantage from disorder: The case of poor language. In C. Marshall (ed.) *Current Issues in Developmental Disorders* (part of the *Current Issues in Developmental Psychology* series) (pp. 125–150). London: Psychology Press.

Sahlén, B., Reuterskiöld-Wagner, C., Nettelbladt, U. and Radeborg, K. (1999) Non-word repetition in children with language impairment – pitfalls and possibilities. *International Journal of Language and Communication Disorders* 34, 337–352.

Seeff-Gabriel, B., Chiat, S. and Dodd, B. (2010) Sentence imitation as a tool in identifying expressive morphosyntactic difficulties in children with severe speech difficulties. *International Journal of Language & Communication Disorders* 45, 691–702.

Seeff-Gabriel, B., Chiat, S. and Roy, P. (2008) *Early Repetition Battery.* London: Pearson Assessment.

Semel, E., Wiig, E. and Secord, W. (1994) *Clinical Evaluation of Language Fundamentals – Revised.* San Antonio, TX: The Psychological Corporation.

Semel E., Wiig, E. and Secord W. (2000) Clinical Evaluation of Language Fundamentals (CELF-IIIUK) (3rd edn). London: Psychological Corporation.

Smith, N. (1973) *The Acquisition of Phonology: A Case Study.* Cambridge: Cambridge University Press.

Stokes, S.F., Wong, A., Fletcher, P. and Leonard, L.B. (2006) Nonword repetition and sentence repetition as clinical markers of specific language impairment: The case of Cantonese. *Journal of Speech, Language, and Hearing Research* 49, 219–236.

Wiig, E., Secord, W. and Semel, E. (1992) *Clinical Evaluation of Language Fundamentals – Preschool.* San Antonio, TX: The Psychological Corporation.

Willis, C.S. and Gathercole, S.E. (2001) Phonological short-term memory contributions to sentence processing in young children. *Memory* 9, 349–63.

4 Assessing Yiddish Plurals in Acquisition: Impacts of Bilingualism

Netta Abugov and Dorit Ravid

The purpose of this study is to assess the acquisition of Yiddish noun plurals among bilingual Ultra-Orthodox Hasidic children in Israel. The Yiddish dialect spoken in the Israeli Hasidic community differs markedly from Standard Yiddish, our major source of knowledge about Yiddish grammar. To establish the baseline of the core nominal lexicon and the plural system IH Yiddish children are exposed to, we first administered a confrontational naming task to 48 IH men and women. Participants were asked to name 95 singular nouns from pictures and provide their plural forms. Results revealed variability in the Israeli Hasidic Yiddish nominal lexicon and plural system, showing how profoundly they both interface with Israeli Hebrew.

Establishing the baseline enabled a good starting point for the developmental study of plural learning by Israeli Hasidic children. A pluralizing task was individually administered to 118 native Yiddish-speaking children and adolescents from the same community. They were asked to provide the plural form of a given singular noun. Results indicate that Yiddish-speaking children display a typical developmental trajectory despite the languages-in-contact situation, in the sense that they learn the plural forms most widely spread in their community including Modern Hebrew singular and plural forms.

Introduction

The current chapter investigates how children deal with variability in the language they are hearing – variability in the choice of marker with individual lemmas, variability in the number of plural markers and variability in the sociolinguistic context in which the language is used. In this context, the current study assesses the native acquisition of Yiddish nouns and noun plurals by children in an Israeli Hasidic (IH) community. Our window on native Yiddish development is the system of noun plurals, a basic morphological category that emerges and develops early on in child language. Plural formation in IH Yiddish is especially interesting, as the system mostly consists of Germanic categories (*kind-er* 'child-ren'), but also contains Hebrew-derived plural markers (*xavéyr-im* 'friend-s') (Laaha *et al.*, 2006; Ravid & Schiff, 2009). These two sources have always been the two major contributors to the Yiddish lexicon and grammar, but the current Israeli-based context has also brought about both contact and friction with Israeli Hebrew, which makes the developmental study of Yiddish plurals even more interesting.

Three assumptions guided us in the current endeavor. First, in general, bilingual learning is assumed to be subject to the relative prominence of the languages under consideration, with the path of acquisition determined by frequency of exposure to each language as well as their reciprocal influence (Gathercole & Hoff, 2007). Second, bilingual development often takes place in 'fluid' situations of variation and change. Thus, whereas young bilinguals generally follow a similar developmental trajectory to that of monolinguals, bilingual learners systematically produce mixed-language or code-switched utterances in different contexts (Paradis *et al.*, 2000) in both lexicon and morphosyntax (Gathercole & Thomas, 2009). A third consideration comes from Nicoladis (2010), namely, that in order for cross-linguistic transfer to occur, the languages may need to share some 'underlying' linguistic structure or conceptualization.

Bearing in mind these key factors, the current chapter aims to (1) find out how Israeli Yiddish-speaking children cope with variability in the input they hear and (2) shed light on the best empirical path to assessment of children's plural productions while taking into account frequency and complexity of the lexical and inflectional input they are exposed to in their speech community.

Israeli Hasidic Yiddish

Yiddish is a Germanic Jewish language that contains a large number of Hebrew words. On the eve of World War II, Yiddish had about 15 million native speakers, most of whom were annihilated in the Holocaust (Harshav, 2006; Katz, 1987; Weinreich, 1980). Yiddish is spoken today by two main groups: the last survivors of pre-Holocaust Eastern Europe, and a rising number of Ultra-Orthodox (UO) Jews (mainly *Hasidim*) worldwide. (Note: We use the term 'Ultra-Orthodox' here. We are aware that Ultra-Orthodoxy is referred to differently in different contexts. Apparently in the US the term is not considered politically correct, whereas in Europe it is; so there are no conventions, but rather preferences.) The exact number of native UO Yiddish speakers today is inaccessible; rough estimates are half a million worldwide (Katz, 2007), but high birth rates and a strong will to maintain a UO life-style may gradually add to these figures. Overall, the Ultra-Orthodox minority is a heterogeneous group regarding its members' countries of origin, study methods, dress-codes, sub-group leaderships and attitudes towards the state of Israel. All these elements interact in the daily life of these groups, and often act as a visible or invisible barrier between them and their secular surroundings (Baumel, 2006; Hason, 2001; Heilman & Friedman, 1991; Levy, 1988; Poll, 1980). Nevertheless, the UO community includes two main groups: *Hasidim*, followers of the Hasidic movement, which is divided into sub-groups such as Belz, Gur and Sanz (often named for the towns and villages in Eastern Europe where they first appeared); and *Misnagdim* (or *Litvish*), historically opponents of the Hasidic movement. Most of today's native Yiddish-speaking population in Israel and worldwide is Hasidic (Katz, 2007).

The segregated Hasidic community in Israel lives in a unique linguistic situation which includes three main languages: Yiddish and Hebrew, two living languages competing as native tongues in a classical bilingual socio-linguistic setting, and *Loshn Koydesh* ('the holy tongue') (LK), which is restricted only to praying and not used for daily communication. The Yiddish-Hebrew balance changes between the different Hasidic groups, so that not all of them speak Yiddish as a native tongue. Israeli Hasidic Yiddish is mostly a spoken language. Reading is engaged in mostly by children, and only extremely conservative schools for girls use Yiddish in writing. Its native speakers do not tend to use dictionaries or grammar books (Goshen-Gottshtein, 1984; Issacs, 1998, 1999; Tannenbaum & Abugov, 2010).

The Hasidic bilingual setting – Yiddish and Hebrew

The establishment of the Hebrew-speaking Israeli state created, for the first time, intensive contact between Israeli Hebrew, the language of the Jewish secular majority, and Yiddish, used for daily communication by the Hasidic population. Israeli Hasidic Yiddish and Hebrew co-exist as two living languages in a language contact situation. Characterizing the type of bilingualism of the IH Yiddish speakers is a complicated task as the balance between Yiddish and Hebrew is inconsistent. Much research is devoted to the different factors affecting bilingualism such as age of exposure and mode of exposure (simultaneous/sequential) (De Houwer, 1995). Yet it is impossible to exclusively relate the IH Yiddish speakers to one sort of factors. Some IH children may be born into a Yiddish-speaking family, and others may be exposed to Yiddish later on. Some children attend a Yiddish-speaking school, whereas others go to a Hebrew-speaking school.

The UO community discriminates Modern Israeli Hebrew from Loshn Koydesh: the former is regarded as the 'spoiled' language of the secular majority, revived by Ben Yehuda 100 years ago, whereas the latter is the holy language of the scriptures - Biblical Hebrew, Mishnaic Hebrew, Post-Biblical Hebrew and Early Rabbinic Hebrew, the language of Rabbinic literature and of rabbis and poskim also in our time. Both languages share the same orthography, but LK employs Ashkenazi pronunciation (Isaacs 1998a, 1999a; Poll 1980).

Weinreich (1972) identifies this contact as 'internal bilingualism', expressing the relationship between two Jewish languages. Although it is perceived as a sacred language that contributes to the Jewish distinctiveness and maintenance (Fishman, 2002), Yiddish constantly intertwines with Hebrew in the Ultra-Orthodox social domain. Fishman (1972) indicates four possible domains that influence language acquisition, maintenance and change: home, neighborhood, education and religion. Whereas *Loshn Koydesh* is used only for religious purposes, the contextual or social division between Yiddish and Hebrew is not apparent. Some Ultra-Orthodox families use Yiddish inside the house and Hebrew outside; in some families only the boys who learn Yiddish in the Yeshiva speak Yiddish, whereas the girls master Hebrew. Some speak Hebrew at home and Yiddish at school. According to Fader (2001, 2006), men and women in the US use Yiddish in different circumstances: Women use Yiddish mostly with small children (baby talk), and men in relation to their sacred study.

Sociolinguistics derives from the study of communities and relates to variability within the community rather than within the individual speaker. Nevertheless, variation within the community originates from variation within the individual speaker, so that the same type of variability can be found at the group level as well as at the individual level (Henry, 1993). Thus, understanding the input at the group level will have an impact on the way in which children from the same community acquire a language. The domain selected for the investigation of this interface is noun plurals, a basic and widely occurring category in the world's languages (Schachter, 1985).

Yiddish noun plurals

Plural formation does not generate a new lexical item, but rather indicates its quantity. Therefore, in morpho-syntactic terms, plural formation is a part of the inflectional system. Yiddish plurals are essentially Germanic in structure, consisting of a set of competing markers. In addition, Yiddish has Hebrew-derived forms, which adds further complexity to the investigation of the system of Yiddish noun plurals.

The point of departure of the current study is the system of noun plurals in Standard Yiddish (SY) which involves suffixation, stem modification or a combination of the two, clearly reflecting the Germanic and the LK Hebrew origins as presented in Reyzen, 1924 and Glasser, 1990. As shown in Table 4.1, the system of noun plurals in Yiddish consists of nine plural markers. Noun

Table 4.1 Plural markers in standard Yiddish

	Example		
Plural marker	Singular	Plural	Gloss
-(e)n	tish	tishn	tables
-s	tate	tates	fathers
-er	kind	kinder	children
Zero	epl	epl	apples
umlaut	kop	kep	heads
umlaut + -er	boim	beimer	trees
-im	xaver	xaveyrim	friends
-es	xale	xales	Shabbat loaves
-(e)x	meydl	meydlex	girls

plurals are formed by five different suffixes *-(e)n*, *-(e)s*, *-er*, *-im*, *-(e)x* or by a *zero* morpheme. Two of these plural markers (*-er* and *zero*) may combine with a stem vowel change whose effect is similar to the umlaut in German. Two plural suffixes, *−im* (-ים) and *-es* (-ת), are of Hebrew origin and take Hebrew nouns. But unlike Hebrew, they do not serve as gender markers.

However, plurals in Hasidic Yiddish do not necessarily adhere to the Standard system; Yiddish noun plurals in the contemporary sociolinguistic setting have not been systematically investigated to date. One seminal work that has appeared, by D. Berman (2007), describes major linguistic phenomena in Israeli UO Yiddish. Berman exemplifies specific morphological changes in the system of noun plurals of Israeli UO Yiddish owing to the influence of Israeli Hebrew. For example, forms such as *shixim* instead of *shix* 'shues'. Berman's examples suggest that UO Yiddish has undergone change owing to the impact of Israeli Hebrew.

The investigated community: Sanz Hasidism in Israel

Sanz Hasidism was founded by the Sanz-Klausenberger Rebbe Halberstam, who lost his family in the Holocaust. His vision was to rebuild the community in Israel and reconstruct the cultural, social, and religious way of life. As has been the case with other Hasidic communities that vanished in the Holocaust, the Rebe gathered around many followers from Poland, Hungary and other Eastern-European communities. Thus, members of the Israeli Sanz Hasidism today come from different geographical origins in Europe, America and Israel.

The city of Natanya is the heart of the community, although there are some families in Jerusalem and Bnei-Barak, and also communities in New York, London and Antwerp. The community in Natanya caters to its 800 families' independent religious lifestyle, including health care systems and a large educational system from infancy to adulthood. All Sanz members are bilingual/multilingual – speaking Yiddish and Hebrew and praying in Loshn Koydesh. Historically speaking, as most Israeli Sanz members are not the descendants of the same people who spoke Yiddish in Polish Nowy Sands, it is impossible to relate their Yiddish to that Yiddish dialect. Yiddish enjoys a higher status than Hebrew and functions as the first language for most of the target families, yet the Sanz educational systems emphasize the role of Yiddish as a spoken language and Hebrew as a written one.

Empirical Investigations

Studying the acquisition of Yiddish noun plurals by Hasidic children has been a complicated task as the plural forms that Israeli Hasidic children were exposed to had never been investigated. Using the system of Standard Yiddish as a baseline would be a serious methodological mistake as it has already been found that this is not the real system used today by the Israeli Ultra-Orthodox community (Berman, 2007).

Therefore, our study included two phases: (1) the Baseline Study and (2) the Developmental Study – both conducted in the same Hasidic community. In (1) our aim was to establish the input children were exposed to, both in the nominal lexicon and in the plural system. This baseline served as the starting point for the second phase of our project – the Developmental Study of plural learning by IH children. In this phase our aim was to trace the route of acquisition of noun plurals in speakers of IH Yiddish in Israel. More specifically, we wanted to determine how children come to acquire the forms that they hear in the input and whether they use the plural forms according to what they hear in the adult language.

Hypotheses

Against this background, we make the following hypotheses: (1) We expect Yiddish-speaking adults to produce a highly variable language with regards to singular nouns and their plural forms. In particular, given the intensive contact with Israeli Hebrew and the underlying features of the two languages, we expect Hebrew to have an impact on singular and plural forms. (2) We expect children to produce the most frequent, regular and consistent forms adults employ so that the distribution of plural forms in children's productions will be similar to those in the adult language (Theakston *et al.*, 2002).

Phase 1 – Obtaining the Baseline

Method
Participants
Participants of the Baseline Study were 48 adults (24 men and 24 women) 21 to 60 years of age (mean age: 32). They were all members of Sanz Hasidism

and lived in Natanya, Israel, and were all married and spoke mostly Yiddish at home.

Procedure

Participants were administered two psycholinguistic tasks based on 95 pictures of everyday objects and abstract items such as a fork, an elephant, a day or a wedding. The first was a Naming Task, for which participants had to provide a lemma or label for each of 95 target items. For example, *xasne* for a wedding or *elefant* or *pil* (the Hebrew word) for *elephant*. The second was a Plural Task, which followed immediately, for which participants had to pluralize the label they had given. The elicitation procedure went as follows: pointing to a picture of a mountain, the researcher first asked (Task 1) *vus is dus?* ('what is this') and the participant replied (for example) *barg* 'mountain'. Then the researcher went on (Task 2) to inquire *'un in loshn rabim* ('and in the plural?') The participant then replied (for example) *berg* 'mountains'. Before the target tasks, participants were given three examples by the researcher, in order to ensure they fully understood the tasks.

Stimuli

Grammatically, the 95 target items were select to represent the nine plural categories in SY (see above in Table 4.1). Content-wise, they represented pragmatic-semantic categories of everyday life. These included animals (e.g. *kac / kec* 'cat-s'), food (*bar / barn* 'pear-s'), body parts (*kop / kep* 'head-s'), clothes (*hemd / hemder* 'shirt-s'), useful objects (*meser / mesers* 'knife-knives'), locations (*shtot / shteyt* 'city-cities'), agent nouns (xaver / xaveyrim 'friend-s'), Jewish terms (*draydl / draydlex* 'dreidel-s'), temporal terms (*shu / shuen* 'hour-s') and events (*xasene /xasenes* 'wedding-s'). All words except ten were elicited in conjunction with a picture representing the given object. Ten of the words were abstract words (*vort / verter* 'word-s'); these were presented to the participants in Hebrew without accompanying pictures, and they were asked to give the Yiddish equivalents.

Results

The naming task

Results of the Naming Task confirmed our expectations by revealing considerable language variation in the lexicons of native Yiddish-speaking adults. Thus, 95 target items yielded 170 lemmas, a mean of 1.8 lemmas per target item. For example, the picture of a king yielded *kéynig, méylex* and *king*. We counted the number of lemmas given to each of the 95 target items as a measure of language variation in the Sanz IH nominal lexicon. The distribution of target items by number of lemmas per item is presented in Figure 4.1.

Figure 4.1 shows that 55% of the target items were designated by a single lemma (e.g. *shtayn* 'stone', *briv* 'letter', *xusn* 'groom'), whereas 45% were labeled with more than one lemma (*shlang* and Hebrew *naxash* for 'snake'; *bal,* English *bol,* Hebrew *kadur* and *tabele* for 'ball').

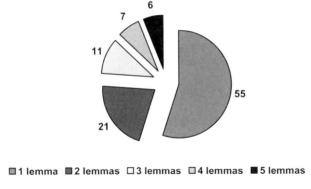

1 lemma   2 lemmas   3 lemmas   4 lemmas   5 lemmas

Figure 4.1 Percentage of lemmas ($N = 170$) per target items ($N = 95$)

In addition, lemmas produced by the adult participants reflect the new sociolinguistic context under the pressure of modern life and Israeli Hebrew, showing that the contemporary Yiddish lexicon is impacted by the Hebrew lexicon. For the 95 items, 21% of the designated lemmas come from Hebrew– for example, *maxshev* for 'computer' and *pil* for 'elephant' – and display a prominent source of variability in the Yiddish lexicon of the adult speakers.

The plural task

Participants were asked to pluralize the lemmas ($N = 170$) they had provided for the target items. For example, *teler* ('plate') was pluralized as *telers* by all study participants. The variegated facets of the Sanz Yiddish nominal lexicon were also apparent in the grammatical system of noun plurals: in sheer numbers, the 170 lemmas entailed 331 plural responses, that is, a mean of 1.9 plural forms per lemma. This distribution is presented in Figure 4.2.

As shown in Figure 4.2, about half of the lemmas had one plural form (e.g. *teler-s* 'plates', *os-oysies* 'letters', *shlisl-ex* 'keys') and half resulted in two

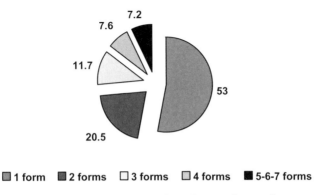

1 form   2 forms   3 forms   4 forms   5-6-7 forms

Figure 4.2 Percentage of plural forms ($N = 331$) per lemmas ($N = 170$)

or more different plural forms (e.g. *bilder* and *bilders* for *bild* 'picture', *trob*, *trobn*, *trobns* and *trobalax* for *trob* 'grape').

We pooled together all 331 plural responses given in the pluralizing task for our analyses and classified them by plural categories. We started by assigning each plural response in our inventory (e.g. *-s, -ex*) into the nine plural categories of Standard Yiddish. However it was soon clear that Sanz Hasidic Yiddish does not entirely adhere to the Standard system. An analysis of adults' plural productions revealed 17 plural markers as presented in Table 4.2.

According to Table 4.2, a new origin of plural marker category - Israeli Hebrew – has emerged (*vilon-ot* 'curtain-s'), which adds to the diversity of the contemporary plural system. In addition, new Germanic plural markers have emerged, all of which are combinations of already existing Standard plural markers. For example, combining Germanic *-n* and *-s* formed the new suffix *–ns* as in *tishns* 'tables' and *shuens* 'hours'. Another example is the combination between *–er* and *–s*, which formed the new suffix *–ers* as in *tishtexers* 'table cloths' and *laybers* 'lions'. More combinations were also produced with the elemental umlaut, adding to the familiar umlaut + *er* the markers umlaut + *ers* as in *mol / maylers* 'mouths', umlaut + *n* as in *tug / tegn* 'days' and umlaut + *s* as in *barg / bergs* 'mountains'. Thus, although the overwhelming

Table 4.2 Plural markers in IH Sanz Yiddish spoken in Israel

Origin	No.	Plural marker	Example	Gloss
Germanic	1	-(e)n	bar-barn	pears
	2*	-ns	zok-zokns	socks
	3	-s	ferd-ferds	horses
	4	-er	tištex-tištexer	table-cloths
	5*	-ers	layb-laybers	lions
	6	Zero	fiš-fiš	fish
	7	Umlaut	kac-kec	cats
	8*	U + ers	boim-baymers	trees
	9*	U + n	barg-bergn	mountains
	10*	U + s	tayp-teyps	tapes
	11	U + -er	kop-keper	heads
	12*	U + ex	kop-kepalax	heads
	13	-ex	benkl-benklex	chairs
Loshn-Koydesh	14	Es	dire-dires	apartments
	15	Im	dokter-doktoyrim	doctors
Israeli Hebrew	16*	Hebrew ot	vilon-vilonot	curtains
	17*	Hebrew im	kadur-kadurim	balls

(*indicates new plural markers which do not occur in Standard Yiddish) majority of Sanz Yiddish plurals are Germanic in character, there have been innovations, including the fact that Israeli Hebrew exerts a clear influence on this system.

Analysis of the frequencies of all plural markers revealed that the most common plural markers in Sanz Yiddish are the -*n* (17.8%) and –*s* (15.1%). The next most common were –*ex* (12.5%) and–*es* (11.8%), closely followed by–*er* (8.7%), umlaut (7.1%) and umlaut + *er* (7.1%), all of which exist in Standard Yiddish. Low-frequency plural markers consist of –*im* and zero (with less than 5 % of the responses for each), showing how unstable their status is. All other low-frequency plural markers are the additional Sanz-specific innovations, with Israeli Hebrew -*im* (3.2%) and –*ot* (2.6%) closely followed by the combined–*ers* (2.5%), and umlaut + *ex* / umlaut + *ers* / umlaut + *n,* umlaut + -*ns,* each receiving less than 1% of the responses. In line with the position that input frequency plays a major role in determining developmental trajectories (Tomasello, 2000), we expected a similar frequency distribution in the children's responses.

In Phase 1 of our study, we thus created a pool of core Yiddish nouns and determined the plural system that applies to them, which provided the baseline for the Developmental Study. Taking into consideration this unfamiliar bilingual setting, we let the adults point the way to the children, in the sense of constituting the input IH speakers are exposed to and establishing the levels of variability in the nominal lexicon and the plural system both in terms of frequency and in terms of complexity.

Phase 2 – The Developmental Study

Obtaining the baseline enabled a valid point of departure for the Developmental Study. In the second phase of our study, we explore how children use the variegated input they are exposed to, and the extent to which the factors of input frequency and linguistic complexity account for plural use in Hasidic Yiddish acquisition.

Method
Participants

The study included 118 native Yiddish-speaking children and adolescents from the same community as the adults. It consisted of 59 girls aged 3, 5, 7, 9, 11, 17 (10 girls for each age group, except for the 7-year-olds, for whom there were nine girls) and 59 boys aged 3, 5, 7, 9, 11, 17 (10 boys for each age group, except for the 7-year-olds, for whom there were nine boys). They all lived in Natanya, Israel, spoke mostly Yiddish at home, and according to teacher and parental report had no developmental or linguistic problems. Additionally, we created a control adult age group ($n = 48$),with participants selected from phase 1. Overall this study consisted of seven age groups: 3–4, 5–6, 7–8, 9–10, 11–12, 17–18 and adults.

Procedure

The Developmental Study is based on a structured elicitation methodology which has been developed and tested within the context of a cross-linguistic project on the acquisition of noun plurals in three Germanic languages (Danish, Dutch and German) compared with Hebrew (Nir-Sagiv *et al.*, 2008). This is an experimental noun plural naming test in the spirit of the classical Wug Test (using real words rather than Pseudo words) (Berko, 1958). The singular form of the noun was introduced (accompanied by pictures, identical to those used in the baseline study), and the participant was asked to provide the plural form of that noun. For example: *es iz du a 'tish' and es zenen du a sax* _____ 'there is a table and there are many _____'.

Stimuli

The task included 60 items, selected from the pool of 95 items created by the Baseline Study. We excluded items that were unsuitable for the Developmental Study, for instance, items that were not familiar to the adults such as 'ostrich' which was labeled by only 29% of the participants (the other 71% did not know what to call it in Yiddish) or 'rabbit' which was labeled only by 17% of the participants (the other 83% did not know what to call it in Yiddish). Five of the items were abstract (*vort-verter* 'word-s', *tug-teg* 'day-s') which were not accompanied by pictures, and were therefore presented to the participants in Hebrew. Seventy-five percent of the items ($n = 45$) were items with only one lemma (singular form) in the phase 1 data and 25% had more than one lemma variation ($n = 15$).

For those items that had more than one singular lemma, we had to decide which of the lemmas to present to the children as the singular form. We decided to present to the child the dominant label for each of the items. For example, although the item 'sock' was designated as both *zok* and *shtrimp* by the adults, we included only the label *zok* as it occurred in 96% of adult responses.

Data analysis – conformity to the adult forms

A major part of this study consisted of examining the development of the plural system in the IH community. In fact, this phase examined to what extent children's plural formation of each noun matched the adult norms. Results of the Baseline Study revealed variation in the plural system so that many of the nouns were given more than one plural form. For example, the singular form *bayzik* ('bike') yielded two adult plural forms: *bayziks* and *bayzikes*. In more stable and robust sociolinguistic contexts the term 'correct' is usually used; for instance, a plural form of a Hebrew or an English singular noun would be acceptable to virtually all literate adults. Here however, we are dealing with language variation and instability and were therefore obliged to approach the issue of attributing the correct plural markers with great caution.

In order to adhere to the variegated input children are exposed to, we first divided all adults' plural productions into 'frequent' and 'infrequent' plural forms (rather than 'correct' and 'incorrect'). Accordingly, upon listing all adult plural responses to all 60 target nouns, we coded plural forms that received less than 15% of the responses for each noun as 'infrequent' plural forms and forms that received more than 15% of the responses as 'frequent'. For example, the target noun *oyg* ('eye') elicited both adult *oygn* (92%) and *oygns* (8%). Whereas *oygn* was coded as a 'frequent' plural form, *oygns* was coded as 'infrequent'.

For all 60 target nouns, we then created a frequency scale for all 'frequent' responses. The scale consisted of three levels of frequency: 'primary', 'secondary' and 'tertiary' frequent plural forms. This classification too was determined by the distribution of adult responses given to the plural form. The most frequent plural form (usually, 80–100% of responses, but the critical factor was that it occurred in the most plurals formed by the adults) was designated 'primary'. These were usually, but not always, items with either one plural form or with a very dominant plural form. For example, the word *bild* ('picture') had only one primary plural form, *bilder,* receiving 94% of the responses. Forms that received 30–40% of the responses were designated Secondary; these were usually, but not always, items with two dominant plural responses. For example, the word *banana* yielded the 'primary' form *bananes*, produced by 62% of the participants, and the 'secondary' form *bananot*, produced by 25% of the participants. Plural forms occurring in 15–20% of the responses were designated as 'tertiary'. For example, the word *bix* 'book' yielded the form *bixlex* (produced by 41% of the participants), which was coded as 'primary', the 'secondary' form *bixer* (produced by 33% of the participants), and the 'tertiary' form *bixn* (produced by 15% of the participants).

Thus, each plural production was first coded as either 'frequent' or 'infrequent'. Following this classification, all frequent responses were coded as 'primary', 'secondary' and 'tertiary'. Overall, the selected 60 items revealed that 60% ($N = 36$) of the nouns had only a 'primary' frequent plural form; 35% ($N = 21$) of the nouns had both 'primary' and 'secondary' plural forms and 5% ($N = 3$) had 'primary', 'secondary' and 'tertiary' frequent plural forms.

Results
Analysis by plural marker

The development of noun plurals among IH Yiddish-speaking children was analyzed taking into account two major factors in bilingual language acquisition: input frequency and linguistic complexity. The most prominent feature of this study is the context in which IH Yiddish is learned: a fluid situation of variation and change, due to the intensive contact with the Modern Hebrew spoken by the secular and non-Hasidic Israeli majority. Establishing the nominal and plural input in the Baseline Study enabled us to assess the actual linguistic features children are exposed to. Bearing in mind the distributions of all 17 plural markers among adults (Table 4.2) we first present their frequencies among children as presented in Figure 4.3.

According to Figure 4.3, the distribution of all 17 plural markers reveals that IH children first learn the most frequent plural markers in the adult community. Thus, Germanic –*n*, *Loshn Koydesh* –*es*, and Germanic –*ex* are the most common plural markers among IH Yiddish-speaking adults as well as children. This serves as another piece of evidence for the role of input in bilingual acquisition. For more detailed analyses see Abugov (2011).

We proceeded by examining the percentages of frequent responses, that is responses that received more than 15% of the responses in the adult usage, according to the six age groups. Figure 4.4 presents the data.

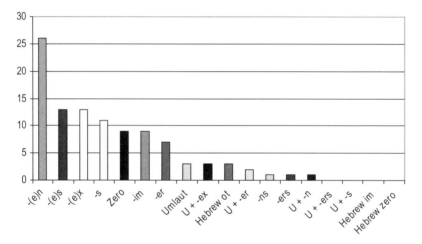

Figure 4.3 Distributions by plural marker

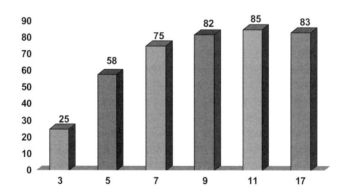

Figure 4.4 Percentage of frequent response by age

Figure 4.4 shows a clear developmental trajectory in producing frequent plural responses, similar to what we see in other languages. Significant differences between age groups were found so that 3-year-olds reach about 25% of usage of forms that were coded as frequent in the adult language – and that is a cut-off point – and 5-year-olds reached about twice that much usage of frequent forms – and that is another cut-off point. By age 7, 75% of the responses were counted as frequent, again a cut-off point. The three oldest groups form one block in which success does not exceed about 80%, reflecting the variation in the community.

Levels of frequency

We now present the analysis of frequent responses (plural forms that received more than 15% of the responses among adults) by age and frequency levels (primary, secondary and tertiary). Participant sex was not significant and was therefore excluded from this analysis. In order to examine frequency levels we conducted a two-way ANOVA of age and frequency levels with repeated measures for frequency levels. Significant differences were found for frequency levels ($F(2,318) = 6690.36$, $p < 0.001$, $\eta p2 = 0.98$) showing that primary responses scored highest (85.99%) followed by secondary (12.05%) and tertiary (1.97%). The interaction of age and frequency levels was also significant ($F(12,318) = 10.48$, $p < 0.001$, $\eta p2 = 0.28$), as depicted in Figure 4.5.

A post-hoc Bonferroni analysis found significant differences at the level of .05, showing that in all age groups, the percentages of primary frequent responses were significantly higher than secondary and tertiary frequent responses. At the age of three, the percentage of primary frequent responses was lower than at all other age groups. Also, at the age of three, the percentage of secondary frequent responses was lower than in all other age

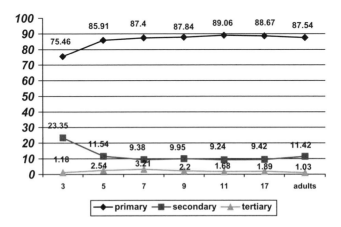

Figure 4.5 Interaction of frequency levels by age

groups. For tertiary frequent responses there were no differences between the age groups.

By way of illustration, the following two tables present the routes of acquisition of the plural forms for two words. Table 4.3 presents the lemma *layter* 'ladder' which, according to the Baseline results, had only one primary plural form: *layters* (100%), and Table 4.4 presents the lemma *dokter* 'doctor', which had two possible frequent plural forms: *dokters* (77%) and *doktoyrim* (21%).

According to Table 4.3, children at the age of 3 already start producing the primary form *layters*, but only at a rate of 20%, together with other plural forms including zero, *-n,-im* and *-ex*. There is a dramatic increase already by age 5 in the use of the primary form. By the age of nine and beyond, all of the children produced the primary plural form exclusively or almost exclusively. According to Table 4.4, despite the variable input, children follow the same forms as the adults, in that the primary response was the most frequent at every age, but its use was initially much lower than among adults. The use of the primary marker and the secondary marker gradually increased, so that by the age of nine and beyond children almost exclusively produced the primary form *dokters* and the secondary form *doktoyrim*, also adhering to the frequency levels in the adult community.

Table 4.3 Route of acquisition – *layter*

Age 3 N = 20	Age 5 N = 20	Age 7 N = 18	Age 9 N = 20	Age 11 N = 20	Age 17 N = 20
layters 20%	layters 65%	layters 78%	layters 100%	layters 95%	layters 100%
laytern 5%	laytern 5%	laytern 22%		laytern 5%	
layterim 5%	layterim 15%				
layter 60%	layter 15%				
laytelex 10%					

Table 4.4 Route of acquisition *dokter*

Age 3* N = 19	Age 5 N = 20	Age 7 N = 18	Age 9 N = 20	Age 11 N = 20	Age 17 N = 20
dokters 26%	dokters 50%	dokters 44%	dokters 60%	dokters 75%	dokters 75%
doktoyrim 10%	doktoyrim 20%	doktoyrim 44%	doktoyrim 40%	doktoyrim 20%	doktoyrim 25%
doktern 5%	doktern 5%	doktern 11%		doktern 5%	
dokter 58%	dokter 25%				

*one participant did not know the plural form

Category of origin
In order to evaluate the influence of the contact between Yiddish and Hebrew in the Hasidic bilingual setting, results were also analyzed according to the three categories of origin: Germanic, LK and Hebrew. Our baseline results have shown that we are investigating the development of noun plurals in a variegated, non-stable situation and that Hebrew is a major player. Table 4.5 presents the distribution of frequent and infrequent results by age group and category of origin.

A three-way ANOVA of age (3, 5, 7, 9, 11, 17, adults) X frequencies (frequent, infrequent) X category of origin (Germanic, *LK*, Hebrew) on the data in Table 4.5 revealed an important effect for category of origin ($F(2,312) = 2468.58$, $p < 0.001$, $\eta_p^2 = 0.94$) so that most responses (both frequent and infrequent) were Germanic in origin ($M = 78.63\%$), followed by *LK* ($M = 15.29\%$), then Hebrew ($M = 6.08$), all significantly different from each other. Two two-way interactions were significant: Age X Category of origin ($F(12,312) = 5.73$, $p < 0.001$, $\eta_p^2 = 0.18$) and Frequency X Category of origin ($F(2,312) = 66.68$, $p < 0.001$ $\eta_p^2 = 0.30$). These interactions were included in the three-way interaction of Age X Frequency X Origin ($F(12, 312) = 5.66$, $p < 0.001$, $\eta_p^2 = 0.18$), depicted in Figure 4.6.

The percentages of frequent and infrequent responses of Germanic origin were higher than the Hebrew and the *LK* origins for all age groups. For the frequent responses, *LK* was higher than Hebrew in all age groups except for the three-year-olds. In addition, for the Germanic origin, there was a greater proportion of less frequent responses than infrequent responses among 11-year-olds, 17-year-olds, and adults. It was also found

Table 4.5 Frequent and infrequent responses by age and category of origin

	Frequent			Infrequent		
	Germanic	LK	Hebrew	Germanic	LK	Hebrew
Age 3	86.62	12.20	1.18	81.57	5.51	10.92
	(10.23)	(9.36)	(2.30)	(11.92)	(10.60)	(6.20)
Age 5	73.58	22.28	4.14	70.69	11.22	18.10
	(5.57)	(5.36)	(2.78)	(15.01)	(13.73)	(8.84)
Age 7	70.98	25.41	3.61	71.82	14.44	13.73
	(4.78)	(4.48)	(1.70)	(22.53)	(19.65)	(12.74)
Age 9	72.55	24.41	3.04	80.33	6.47	13.21
	(2.62)	(2.25)	(1.29)	(17.15)	(12.84)	(12.90)
Age 11	73.30	24.08	2.62	90.58	5.47	3.96
	(2.53)	(2.37)	(1.10)	(13.81)	(8.20)	(9.41)
Adults	75.60	21.80	2.60	89.55	10.45	0
	(5.11)	(4.50)	(1.60)	(20.03)	(20.03)	(0)

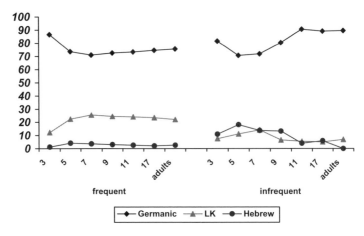

Figure 4.6 Interaction of age group, frequency and origin

that for *LK* origin plurals, there were more uses of frequent forms than infrequent forms among the 9-year-olds, 11-year-olds, 17-year-olds, and adults. Finally, for the infrequent responses, the use of Germanic origin forms was higher among 11-year-olds, 17-year-olds, and adults than among 5- and 7-year-olds, and the use of Hebrew origin forms was higher at the age of 5 than among adults.

Discussion

The general framework of the current study was the context in which IH Yiddish is learned: a fluid situation of variation and change and intensive contact with the Modern Hebrew spoken by the secular and non-Hasidic Israeli majority. Establishing the nominal and plural input in the Baseline Study enabled us to assess the actual linguistic features children were exposed to. Two major factors in bilingual language acquisition were taken into account: input frequency of lemmas and plurals in the data of this study (based on the Baseline Study) and linguistic complexity of Yiddish as well as Hebrew plural markers. It is thus interesting to see that, in line with Paradis *et al.* (2000), Yiddish acquisition in the Israeli Hasidic context on the one hand displayed a similar developmental trajectory to that of monolinguals, and on the other hand incorporates Modern Hebrew lexical items in the production of morphological constructions (*vilon-ot* 'curtain-s').

In terms of input frequency, an interesting finding emerged from the analysis of frequent responses by age and frequency levels – primary, secondary and tertiary. Yiddish-speaking children display a typical developmental trajectory despite the languages-in-contact situation, in the sense that they learn the plural forms most widespread in their community. We found that in all age groups, the percentages of primary frequent responses were significantly higher than secondary and tertiary frequent responses. For example, most participants in all age groups produced the primary form *dokters* 'doctors' rather than the secondary form *doktoyrim*. Thus, the view by which the path of acquisition is determined by frequency of exposure to each language as well as their reciprocal influence (Gathercole & Hoff, 2007) plays a major role in explaining the way these children learn the three frequency levels.

The importance of input frequency and linguistic complexity were further supported by our analysis according to the three plural origins – Germanic, *LK* and Israeli Hebrew. We took into account both frequent and infrequent plural responses, that is, also those plural forms not considered as primary, secondary, or tertiary. Results showed that Germanic plurals constituted the majority of plural markers and are distributed evenly across frequent and infrequent plural responses. More *LK* forms occurred in the frequent responses, while Modern Israeli Hebrew cropped up in the infrequent responses, indicating a new source of language change in Yiddish which nonetheless does not threaten the predominance of the Germanic plural markers.

Taking this idea further, as suggested by Nicoladis *et al.* (2010), although the IH Yiddish plural system exhibits a stable Germanic core together with elements from *LK*, Modern Hebrew is found to be the key factor differentiating the Hasidic Yiddish plural system from the Standard system. It may well be the case that the 'older', *LK* components in IH Yiddish facilitate the introduction of newer Modern Hebrew elements constituting its 'underlying structure in both of a bilingual's languages' (Nicoladis *et al.*, 2010: 346).

Conclusion

This chapter sheds light on the way to assess language acquisition in cases of multilingual and sociolinguistically fluid language input. It shows how closely children follow what they hear despite variability in the input. The developmental perspective taken in this study allowed us to analyze processes of language variation that were found in the Baseline and observe how they are reflected in younger age groups.

Yiddish in the last century has gone through so many trials: changing its location (in and outside Europe), decreasing and increasing in number of native speakers, changing its context into a religious setting, exposing itself to contact with other languages etc. The current study shows that Hasidic Yiddish in Israel is still undergoing major changes, still adapting to its new setting and context. Thus, the fluid nature of Yiddish requires researchers to understand the overall situation of Yiddish not only among children, but also among adults, using organized systematic research methods. In the current study, had we looked only at the results of the Developmental Study, we would not have understood the true psycholinguistic picture. The Baseline revealed a very fluid picture in which there were different lemmas, different plurals for each lemma, multiple plural markers and combinations, and this allowed us to make sense of the children's performance. The psycholinguistic reality of Israeli Hasidic Yiddish plurals is under flux, and language frequency and complexity were here seen to be major factors in the assessment of Yiddish-Hebrew native speakers.

Acknowledgment

The first author is grateful to the Azrieli Foundation for the award of an Azrieli Fellowship

References

Abugov, N. (2011) Child and adult noun plurals in Israeli Yiddish: A psycholinguistic study in the Hasidic community. Doctoral dissertation. Tel Aviv University, Israel.

Baumel, S.D. (2006) *Sacred Speakers – Language and Culture among the Haredim in Israel.* New York: Berghahn Books.

Berman, D. (2007) Shimur ve-tmura bayiddish haharedit be-Israel [Maintenance and change in Haredi Yiddish in Israel] Doctoral dissertation. Hebrew University,Israel.

Berko, J. (1958) The child's learning of English morphology. *Word* 14, 150–177.

De Houwer, A. (1995) Bilingual language acquisition. In P. Fletcher and B. MacWhinney (eds) *The Handbook of Child Language* (pp. 219–250) Oxford, UK: Blackwell.

Fader, A. (2001) Literacy, bilingualism and gender in a Hasidic community. *Linguistics and Education* 12 (3), 261–283.

Fader, A. (2006) Learning faith: Language socialization in a Hasidic community. *Language in Society* 35 (2), 207–229.

Fishman, J.A. (1972) Domains and the relationship between micro- and macro-sociolinguistics. In J.J. Gumperz and D. Hymes (eds) *Directions in Sociolinguistics* (pp. 435–453). New York & London: Holt, Rinehart and Winston.

Fishman, J.A. (2002) The holiness of Yiddish: Who says Yiddish is holy and why? *Language Policy* 1, 123–141.

Gathercole, V.C.M. and Hoff, E. (2007) Input and the acquisition of language: Three questions. In E. Hoff and M. Shatz (eds) *The Handbook of Language Development* (pp. 107–127). London: Blackwell Publishers.

Gathercole, V.C.M. and Thomas, E.M. (2009) Bilingual first-language development: Dominant language takeover, threatened minority language take-up. *Bilingualism: Language and Cognition* 12, 213–237.

Glasser, P.D. (1990) A distributed approach to Yiddish inflection. Doctoral dissertation, Colombia University, United States.

Goshen-Gottstein, E.R. (1984) Growing up in 'Geula': Socialization and family living in an ultra-orthodox Jewish subculture. PhD, Bar Ilan University, Ramat-Gan.

Hason, S. (2001) Territories and identities in Jerusalem. *Geo Journal* 53, 311–332.

Heilman, S.C. and Friedman, M. (1991) Religious fundamentalism and religious Jews: The case of the Haredim. In M.E. Marty and R.S. Appleby (eds) *Fundamentalisms Observed* (pp. 197–264). Chicago/London: University of Chicago Press.

Henry, A. (1993) Variability and language acquisition. *Proceedings of the 25th Annual CLRF* (pp. 280–286).

Herzog, M.I. (1965) *The Yiddish Language in Northern Poland: Its Geography and History.* Bloomington, IN: Indiana University.

Isaacs, M. (1998) Yiddish in the Orthodox communities of Jerusalem. In D. Kerler (ed.) *Politics of Yiddish* (pp. 85–96). Walnut Creek, CA: AltamiraPress.

Isaacs, M. (1999) Contentious partners: Yiddish and Hebrew in Haredi Israel. *International Journal of the Sociology of Language* 138, 101–121.

Katz, D. (1987) *Grammar of the Yiddish Language.* London: Duckworth.

Katz, D. (2004, 2007) *Words on Fire: The Unfinished Story of Yiddish.* New York: Basic Books.

Kerler, D.B. (1999) *The Origins of Modern Literary Yiddish.* Oxford: Oxford University Press.

Kleine, A. (2003) Standard Yiddish. *Journal of the International Phonetic Association* 33 (2), 261–265.

Köpcke, K-M. (1998) The acquisition of plural marking in English and German revisited: Schemata versus rules. *Journal of Child Language* 25, 293–319.

Krogh, S. (2007) Zur Diachronie der nominalen Pluralbildung im Ostjiddischen. In H. Fix (ed.), *Beiträge zur Morphologie* (pp. 259–285). Germanisch, Baltisch, Ostseefinnisch. University Press of Southern Denmark, Odense.

Laaha, S., Ravid, D., Korecky-Croll, K. and Laaha, G. (2006) Early noun plurals in German: Regularity, productivity or default? *Journal of Child Language* 33, 271–302.

Lincoff, B. (1963) A study in inflectional morphologic development: Old and middle Yiddish. Doctoral dissertation, New York University

Mark, Y. (1978) *Gramatik fun der yiddisher klal-shprakh [A Grammar of Standard Yiddish].* New York: Congress for Jewish Culture.

Nicoladis, E., Rose, A. and Foursha-Stevenson, C. (2010) Thinking for speaking and cross-linguistic transfer in preschool bilingual children. *International Journal of Bilingual Education and Bilingualism* 13 (3), 345–370.

Nir-Sagiv, B., Zwilling, H., Abugov, N., Ravid, D., Laaha, S., Korecky-Kröll, K., Rehfeldt, K., Kjaerbaek Hansen, L. and Basbøll, H. (2008) Why are noun plurals hard to acquire? A multi-task approach. Cross-sectional naturalistic elicitations: Scripts and conversations in Hebrew, Austrian German, and Danish. *Paper presented at the XI International Congress for the Study of Child Language (IASCL),* Edinburgh, UK.

Poll, S. (1980) The sacred-secular conflict in the use of Hebrew and Yiddish among the Ultra-Orthodox Jews of Jerusalem. *International Journal of the sociology of Language* 24, 109–125.

Rayfield, J.R. (1970) *The Language of a Bilingual Community.* The Hague: Mouton.

Ravid, D. (2004) Later lexical development in Hebrew: Derivational morphology revisited. In R.A. Berman (ed.) *Language Development across Childhood and Adolescence: Psycholinguistic and Crosslinguistic Perspectives* (pp. 53–82). Amsterdam: Benjamins.

Ravid, D. and Schiff, R. (2009) Morpho-phonological categories of noun plurals in Hebrew: A developmental study. *Linguistics* 47, 45–63.

Reyzen, Z. (1924) Gramatisher min in Yiddish [Grammatical gender in Yiddish] Yiddishe filologye 1 (pp. 11–22, 2–2, 180–192, 4–6, 303–322).

Schachter, P. (1985) Part of speech systems. In T. Shopen (ed.) *Language Typology and Syntactic Description,* vol. 1: *Clause Structure* (pp. 3–61). Cambridge: Cambridge University Press.

Tannenbaum, M. and Abugov, N. (2010) The legacy of the linguistic fence: Linguistic patterns among Ultra-Orthodox Jewish girls. *Heritage Language Journal* 7 (1), 74–90.

Tomasello, M. (2000) Do young children have adult syntactic competence? *Cognition* 74, 209–253.

Volf, M. (1977) Fonologishe protsesn by mertsol formatsia [Phonological processes in plural forms] In S. Werses, N. Rotenstreich and C. Shmeruk (eds) *Dov Sadan Book* (pp. 120–137). HaKibutz Hameuhad, Israel.

Weinreich, M. (1972) Internal bilingualism in Ashkenaz. In I. Howe and E. Greenberg (eds) *Voices from the Yiddish* (pp. 279–288). Ann Arbor: University of Michigan Press.

Weinreich, M. (1980) *History of the Yiddish language*. Chicago and London: The University of Chicago Press.
Weinreich, U. (1977) *Modern English-Yiddish, Yiddish-English Dictionary*. New York: Yivo. Institute for Jewish Research.
Zaretski, A. (1926) *Praktishe Yidishe gramatik*. Moscow: Farlag 'shul un buxn'.
Zaretski, A. (1929) *Yiddishe gramatik: naye ibergebete oysgabe*. Vilna.

5 Measuring Grammatical Knowledge and Abilities in Bilinguals: Implications for Assessment and Testing

Rocío Pérez-Tattam,
Virginia C. Mueller Gathercole,
Feryal Yavas and Hans
Stadthagen-González

This chapter focuses on the assessment of grammatical knowledge and abilities in bilinguals. It examines bilingual performance in Spanish and English on a test of receptive grammatical knowledge and compares it to monolingual performance, discussing possible interpretations of the similarities and differences between them and ramifications for assessment. The linguistic data come from early bilingual adults who have grown up in the United States, in Florida, and who acquired both languages simultaneously or started acquiring their second language early in life. Exposure to the two languages differed across groups in relation to their 'origin home language' when they were children: Spanish and English at Home ('ESH'), Only Spanish at Home ('OSH') and L1 Spanish-Early L2 English ('L1S- L2E'). The results show differential performance by home language and level of SES (with the father's profession as a proxy) in Spanish, but not in English. This is interpreted in terms of differential exposure to English vs. Spanish, and in the wider context of the sociolinguistic situation in Florida and more generally the United States. General implications for the assessment and testing of bilinguals for linguistic abilities, and more specific implications for the design of assessment instruments for grammatical knowledge are discussed.

Background and Rationale

Grammatical knowledge is central to the use of and proficiency in a language. Grammatical forms and the rules that govern them are at the heart of curriculum design, material preparation, instruction and classroom assessment for many foreign language educators (Purpura, 2004). However, much of the research on grammar assessment and testing focuses on second or foreign language learning contexts, where learners are instructed explicitly and for whom differences are expected relative to monolingual usage. Our focus here is on cases in which learners have acquired both languages from early on, with (mostly) implicit grammatical knowledge of both of their languages, like monolingual native speakers; their knowledge may show different degrees of attainment in either or both languages, like second or foreign language learners, but those differences may be much more covert than in the case of second language learners.

Early bilingual learners show 'distributed' knowledge of their two languages (Grosjean, 1998; Oller & Pearson, 2002), i.e. they may be more proficient in some ways in one language and in other ways in the other language. This is because language acquisition is dependent on input in the given language and interaction with interlocutors speaking that language in real-world contexts (Gathercole & Hoff, 2007; Tomasello, 2003), and exposure to the two languages can occur in distinct contexts, sometimes including distinct interlocutors, distinct socio-cultural contexts and distinct educational contexts. In addition, early bilingual learners in a bilingual community acquire their languages in the wider sociolinguistic context in which their two languages may enjoy different status as a majority vs. minority language in the community.

Furthermore, there is strong evidence that knowledge of one language might affect the use of the other language in bilinguals (e.g. Hernandez *et al.*, 1994; Kilborn & Ito, 1989; Paradis, 2000); thus, some have suggested, under certain conditions, there can be carry-over from one language to the other (e.g. Cook, 2003; Döpke, 2000; Gathercole *et al.*, 2005; Kupisch, 2007; Müller & Hulk, 2001). As put forward by Grosjean (1985, 1989, 1998), the interaction between the two languages causes bilinguals to develop competencies that are different from those of the corresponding monolinguals; therefore, bilinguals might not be equally proficient in all language skills for both languages.

Regarding assessment, these facts have implications for testing bilinguals, for general linguistic abilities as well as grammatical knowledge. The first implication is that for a complete assessment of bilinguals' general language abilities, speakers should be tested in both of their languages. Testing in only one language provides an incomplete and potentially skewed picture of the bilingual's knowledge (Pearson & Fernández, 1994; Pearson *et al.*, 1993). A second implication is that, even if tested in both languages, the tests should be normed on bilinguals, not monolinguals (alone) (Gathercole *et al.*,

2008). Because bilinguals' exposure to and organization of language can be different from those of monolinguals, their performance, when probed in either language, can be expected to differ in sometimes subtle ways from that of monolinguals.

It is worth stressing that bilinguals are far from the exception among speakers of the world's languages. In the United States, one of the main immigrant languages is Spanish, which is reported to be the main language spoken at home by approximately 35.5 million people aged 5 or older (2009 Selected Social Characteristics, United States Census Bureau). The same survey reports that 12.4% of the US population speaks Spanish or a Spanish Creole, and that 54.3% of the Spanish-speaking populations also speak English 'very well'. The assessment of Spanish/English bilinguals who have grown up in the United States, learning Spanish (the minority language) at home and English (the majority language) in the wider community, from birth or early in life, is key to understanding their performance along the path towards adulthood.

For a clear picture of language abilities in bilinguals, any assessment should take both of their languages into consideration. The results of such tests might not only be important for the individuals involved, but can also have important implications for language policy and education. It is typical for bilinguals to be assessed only in English (or the relevant dominant language), and they are measured against monolingual standards or language proficiency targets set by legislation (e.g. No Child Left Behind Act, see Caldas, this volume). Although there is a provision in No Child Left Behind that allows states to test English Language Learners in their native language for up to three years, assessments in languages other than English are either unavailable or not aligned with state standards. Some of the tests used merely translate English language tests. And for students who are taught primarily in English and have limited literacy in their native language, native language testing is not appropriate (Crawford, 2004). As a result, language skills in bilinguals are often underestimated.

In this chapter we examine the efficacy of the use of two parallel tests for the assessment of bilinguals' receptive proficiency in their two languages, here Spanish and English. We focus on a population that has had optimal opportunities for acquiring their two languages – end-state, highly educated bilingual adults in the Miami setting. We were interested in knowing whether even under optimal conditions one might be able to discern any differences across sub-groups in their performance on their two languages. We examine monolinguals' and bilinguals' performance on a receptive grammar task in each of their languages, and we explore the roles of language exposure and of extra-linguistic factors on performance. The protocols used in this study compare bilinguals' abilities for similar grammatical structures in the two languages, allowing us to tap into a fine-grained view of bilinguals' performance (in this case, at the end-state). Exposure to the two languages is controlled in relation to the adults' 'origin home language' (the language(s) spoken in the home when the adult was a child, see Gathercole, 2007), and the influence of socio-economic status (SES) is probed through the use of an extensive background questionnaire.

The Study

In order to gain a relatively global assessment of children's and adults' abilities in English and Spanish in the Miami context, we developed two parallel receptive grammar tasks. The focus was to explore abilities on a series of morphosyntactic forms in English and Spanish that are functionally similar across the two languages. (These tests were designed primarily to elicit background information on the language proficiency of participants for a number of experimental tasks, not reported here.)

Method

Stimuli

The two grammar tasks elicit comprehension data by means of a forced-choice picture task. These tasks are based on earlier versions that had been developed for a project dealing with the acquisition of English and Welsh in bilingual children (Gathercole et al., this volume; Gathercole et al., in press). For Welsh, normative assessments were not previously available (see Gathercole et al., this volume), and the goal was to develop two tests that would probe children's and adults' abilities on comparable structures in their two languages. As in the DASG (Developmental Assessment of Spanish Grammar, Toronto, 1976), the DSS (Developmental Sentence Scoring) for English (Lee & Canter, 1971), the TROG (Test of the Reception of Grammar, Bishop, 1979), and the TROG-2 (Psychological Corporation Ltd, 2003), the goal was to collect responses on items covering a wide range of grammatical structures.

The Spanish version of the grammar task was adapted from those developed for Welsh and English. The form of the test was as follows.

(1)   Linguistic forms: Thirteen major structure types were tested. The 13 types, with example sentences from English and Spanish, are shown in Table 5.1. As bilinguals were being tested in both languages, two versions of the Spanish and English tests (version A and version B) were prepared, so that each participant had a different version of the test for each language. In each version, each grammatical structure type was tested with three trials. The lexical items used for versions A and B were the same, except that their occurrence was distributed across distinct trials and structures.

(2)   Nonlinguistic stimuli: Each sentence was paired with a set of four pictures shown simultaneously on a computer screen. These were labeled A, B, C and D. One was the target, expected response, and the other three distractors.

Table 5.1 Structure types tested

Structure type	English sample sentence	Spanish sample sentence
Active	The boy kissed the girl	El niño besó a la niña
Comparative	The egg is lower than the hoop	El huevo está más bajo que el anillo
Superlative	The purple elephant is biggest	El elefante morado es el más grande
Negation	The goats aren't eating	Las cabras no están comiendo
Passive (truncated)	The lion was bitten	El león fue mordido
Time Conjunctions (*before, after, until*)	Before the teacher fell, she took her hat off	Antes de que se cayese, la maestra se quitó el sombrero
Present Perfect/ Past Simple	The boats have sunk	Los barcos se hundieron en el mar
Future	The ducks will jump over the rock	Los patos van a saltar la roca
SS Relative Clauses	The woman who pinched the clown had a box	La mujer que pellizcó al payaso tenía una maleta
OS Relative Clauses	A doctor pushed the princess who was holding a stick	El medico empujó a la princesa que llevaba un bastón
SO Relative Clauses	The donkey that a cow held had a purple tail	El burro al que levantó la vaca tenía una cola morada
Universal or Exhaustive Quantification (*every, both*)	Every princess is on a tractor	Cada princesa está en un tractor
Partial or Non-Exhaustive Quantification (*some, not all*)	Some of the dancers are wearing dresses	Algunas de las bailarinas llevan falda

Participants

A total of 93 bilingual adults were tested for the Spanish and the English grammar tasks. Control groups of English monolingual adults (Mon E) ($N = 24$) and Spanish monolingual adults (Mon S) ($N = 24$) were also tested. The bilinguals were recruited in the Miami area, and most of them were college or graduate students at the time of testing (mean age 22.5, range 18 to 60 years; 20 male, 73 female). The English monolinguals (mean age 31.7, range 18 to 60 years; 12 male, 12 female) were also recruited in the Miami area, and the Spanish monolinguals (mean age 31.8, range 18 to 50 years; 8 male, 16 female) were recruited in Managua, Nicaragua.

In addition to the test stimuli, participants were given a language background questionnaire, which elicited information on their linguistic and educational backgrounds. Through this questionnaire, information on environmental factors such as differential exposure to the languages or the majority language in the community was obtained.

The bilinguals were subdivided by origin home language, as reported in the language assessment questionnaire, and according to whether they had been born in the United States or not. This resulted in three (origin) home language groups: Spanish and English at Home ('ESH') ($N = 32$), Only Spanish at Home ('OSH') ($N = 36$) and L1 Spanish-Early L2 English ('L1S-L2E') ($N = 25$). Participants in the ESH and OSH groups were all born in the United States. Participants in the L1S-L2E group moved to the US between the ages of 1;00 and 12;00 and began learning English once in the US In short, the bilinguals taking part in the study had spent all or most of their lives in the US. All had received their education in English.

Procedure

Participants were tested in both languages, on separate occasions. At the beginning of each session, the experimenter read the following instructions in the relevant language:

English version:

'I'm going to say some things and show you some pictures. Some of the things I say are about people, some are about animals and some are about things. I want you to listen and look at the pictures. Each time, I'll show you four pictures. I want you to look at the pictures carefully and choose the one that matches the sentence best. Sometimes, there will be more than one picture that fits, but choose the *best* one. Take your time and if you want to hear the sentence again, you can'.

Participants started out with five practice trials, unrelated to the structures of interest, to familiarize them with the procedure before moving on to the experimental trials. All verbal stimuli were presented aurally. Participants were asked to indicate their choice by saying the letter corresponding to their choice out loud. The experimenter marked their choice on an answer sheet.

Results

Each type of grammatical structure was scored for number correct (out of three). Performance in the two languages was first analyzed separately, to include the monolinguals for each language in the analyses.

English

Performance on English by structure type and home language is shown in Figure 5.1. An ANOVA in which structure type and home language were treated as variables showed no main effect of home language (F (3, 110) = 0.39, p = 0.762), but there was a significant main effect of type of structure (F (12, 1320) = 16.29, p < 0.001). Post-hoc comparisons revealed that the structures largely fell into two groups, with poorer performance on the future, SO relative clauses, the superlative, time conjunctions and SS relative clauses, on the one hand, than on all the other structures (except that the SS relatives also differed from the SO relatives, p = 0.001), on the other, all pairwise comparisons ps ≤ 0.041; and performance on the passive higher than not only these items but also the comparative, OS relatives, and universal quantification, all ps ≤ 0.045. Performance on OS relatives was also lower than on the present perfect and partial quantification, ps ≤ 0.047. There was no significant two-way interaction of home language and structure.

In sum, although there was differential performance across structures, the results indicate that bilinguals across the three origin home language groups and the English monolinguals performed equivalently. Their performance was high: total mean scores for bilinguals and monolinguals averaged 36.59 correct (out of 39).

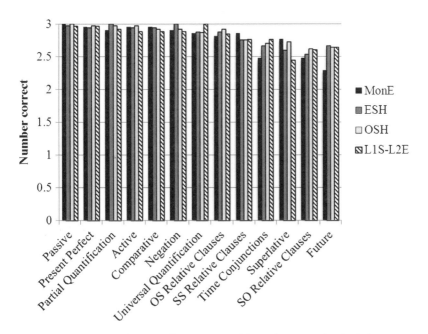

Figure 5.1 Performance by type of structure and home language (ENGLISH)

Spanish

Performance on Spanish by structure type and home language is shown in Figure 5.2. An ANOVA in which structure type and home language were treated as variables showed main effects of home language (F (3, 113) = 4.63, p = 0.004) and of type of structure (F (12, 1356) = 57.93, p < 0.001), and a significant two-way interaction of type of structure and home language (F (36, 1356) = 4.04, p < 0.001). Post-hoc comparisons across language groups revealed that the Spanish monolinguals performed significantly lower than the L1S-L2E bilinguals (p < 0.001) and the OSH bilinguals (p = 0.038), and the ESH bilinguals performed significantly lower than the L1S-L2E bilinguals (p = 0.014). (Mon S: mean score = 33.25; ESH: mean = 34.22; OSH: mean = 34.69; L1S-L2E: mean = 35.96).

Post-hoc comparisons across structures revealed that the structures fell into four groups. Performance on the SO relative clauses was the poorest of all structures, all pairwise comparisons ps < 0.001. Performance on universal quantification, the superlative, the past simple, time conjunctions, and SS relative clauses was next best, and significantly poorer than all the other structures, all ps ≤ 0.041; the next best performance was on the future and OS relatives, which showed significantly lower scores than negation, active, passive, partial quantification, and the comparative, all ps ≤ 0.023.

Simple effects analyses indicated that home language groups differed in performance on a number of structures. For some of these, higher performance corresponded with greater experience with Spanish: on SO relative

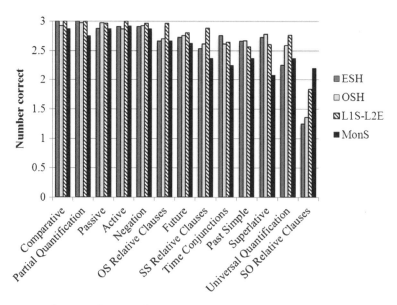

Figure 5.2 Performance by type of structure and home language (SPANISH)

clauses (F (3, 113) = 8.11, $p < 0.001$), the Mon S had higher scores than the ESH and OSH bilinguals, $p = 0.001$, $p = 0.002$, respectively; on universal quantification (F (3, 113) = 3.60, $p = 0.016$), L1S-L2E had higher scores than ESH bilinguals, $p = 0.031$. For others, however, bilinguals showed higher scores than the monolinguals: On the superlative (F (3, 113) = 9.21, $p < 0.001$), Mon S showed lower scores than ESH, OSH, and L1S-L2E bilinguals, all ps ≤ 0.012; on time conjunctions (F (3, 113) = 2.95, $p = 0.036$), Mon S were lower than ESH bilinguals, $p = 0.046$; on SS relatives (F (3, 113) = 3.61, $p = 0.016$, Mon S were lower than L1S-L2E bilinguals, $p = 0.021$; and on partial quantification (F (3, 113) = 5.59, $p = 0.001$), Mon S scored lower than the three groups of bilinguals, all ps ≤ 0.016 (all comparisons Scheffe's multiple comparisons).

These results indicate that on some structures, groups with less exposure to Spanish performed less well than those with more exposure. Thus, for example, on SO structures such as *La bailarina a la que llamó la niña tenía un anillo* 'A dancer that the girl called had a ring', the bilinguals with less exposure to Spanish (ESH, OSH) performed less well than the Spanish monolinguals. An interesting component of these relative clauses in Spanish is the occurrence of the object marker *a* when the object is human, as in *La bailarina [a la que llamó la niña] tenía un anillo*. Without the *a*, such a sentence could be taken as a parenthetical remark with *la* as the subject: *La bailarina – la que llamó...* 'The ballerina – the one who called the girl – has a ring'. We speculate that the difference in performance between the monolinguals, on the one hand, and the OSH and ESH participants, on the other, has to do with attention to or processing of this marker.

For other structures, the Spanish monolinguals seemed to perform at a lower rate than some of the bilinguals. For example, on the superlative, Spanish monolinguals performed significantly lower than every bilingual group, and on time conjunctions, the monolinguals had lower scores than the ESH bilinguals. At first glance, these results seem surprising; but on closer examination of the data, these results appear to reveal important differences in the way in which monolingual Spanish speakers and their bilingual counterparts process these forms. In relation to the superlative, for example, there are some crucial differences between the English and Spanish structures that might explain the difference between the Spanish monolinguals' performance and the bilinguals' performance. In English, there is a clear dichotomy between the superlative and the comparative: the superlative is derived from inflecting adjectives with the suffix *–est*, as in *The policeman is fattest*; the comparative is formed with the suffix *–er*. In Spanish, the two are essentially the same structure; the only difference is that the superlative carries the definite article *el/la*. Thus, the comparative and superlative both use *más* 'more' before the adjective, as in *El policía es más gordo*; the superlative simply adds the article: *El policía es el más gordo*. Thus, the superlative in Spanish is not as contrastive with the comparative as it is in English.

We speculate that bilinguals might be using their knowledge of the English comparative-superlative contrast to interpret Spanish structures. If so, this would be a case in which we can observe influence of one language (here, English) on the interpretation of the other (Spanish) (in this case, a sort of 'hyper-grammaticization').

In relation to time conjunctions, if we look at the performance within the different trials, the Spanish monolinguals had comparatively more difficulties with the structures that included the conjunction *hasta* 'until' (e.g. *la pinza no se cayó hasta que despegó el avión* 'the peg did not fall until the plane took off'). In contrast, the bilinguals' performance in Spanish was uniform across all three time conjunctions (*antes* 'before', *después* 'after', *hasta* 'until'). We speculate that the differences in performance have to do, again, with English vs. Spanish structure. In contrast with English *until*, which has only a temporal reading, the Spanish preposition *hasta* has both a temporal and a spatial reading. The temporal reading is equivalent to *until* (*Me quedé hasta el viernes* 'I stayed until Friday'). The spatial reading is roughly equivalent to *up to* (*El agua me llega hasta las rodillas* 'the water comes up to my knees'). We speculate that Spanish monolinguals might have been influenced by both readings when processing the sentences involving *hasta*. In contrast, bilinguals might have been using their knowledge of the narrower application of *until* (with only a temporal reading) and applying this to Spanish. If so, this is another case in which the bilinguals' interpretation of Spanish, in this case especially the ESH bilinguals, is influenced by their knowledge of English.

Such results concerning the interpretation, e.g. of the superlative with *más* and time conjunctions including *hasta* mean that Spanish monolinguals' understanding of these grammatical forms may be more flexible or less specific than is relevant to the understanding of the comparable forms in English. The more specific meanings associated with the English structures may be being used by the bilinguals to interpret the Spanish forms. The superlative and time conjunctions appear, therefore, to be not completely equivalent in Spanish and English, and the responses that they elicit show subtle distinctions. The inclusion of forms such as these in a test of this kind may be useful, in that they can reveal subtle differences in processing, but their inclusion in a normalization of such a test would have to be weighed carefully.

In sum, the results for Spanish indicate differential performance in bilinguals across the three origin home language groups and the Spanish monolinguals, as well as across structures. On the whole, performance among the bilinguals was high, with the total mean scores for bilinguals averaging 34.53 correct (out of 39), but the ESH bilinguals performed significantly lower than the L1S-L2E bilinguals. Performance of the bilinguals relative to the monolinguals, however, revealed differential performance on certain structures across the groups: the Mon S speakers had higher scores on the SO relatives, perhaps revealing better processing of the accusative marker *a*; and the Mon S speakers showed different interpretations for the superlative and the time conjunctions than the bilingual speakers, which we have suggested may correspond to the bilinguals' application of English-like interpretations within the Spanish context.

Comparison of performance in English and Spanish

In order to compare bilingual participants' relative language abilities in their two languages, correlational analyses of scores on the two grammar tasks were calculated. The overall correlations in performance on the two grammar tasks are relatively high, both for all bilinguals pooled together ($r = 0.43$, $p < 0.001$) and for every separate bilingual group: L1S-L2E ($r = 0.65$, $p < 0.001$), ESH ($r = 0.40$, $p = 0.025$) and OSH ($r = 0.42$, $p = 0.011$). See the scatter plot in Figure 5.3, which visually shows the performance by the bilinguals on English and Spanish. This suggests that bilinguals who perform well in one language tend to perform well in the other. This is consistent with the data on linguistic abilities in Welsh/English bilingual children presented by Gathercole *et al.* (this volume): children's abilities in their two languages become more similar and more highly correlated with age, and earlier for grammatical abilities than for vocabulary abilities. That is, by the teenage

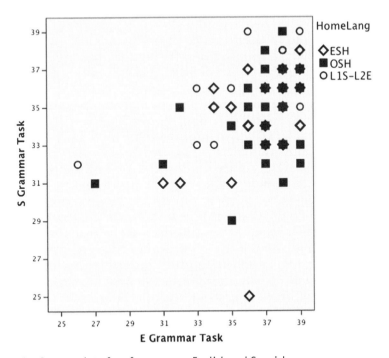

Figure 5.3   Scatter plot of performance on English and Spanish

years and adulthood, the evidence shows general parity of performance across a bilingual's two languages, at least in sociolinguistic contexts of widespread community bilingualism such as Miami and North Wales.

Are these high correlations related to direct links across structures, or are they indicative of a more general level of language proficiency in individuals? To answer this, we can look at performance on the individual sub-structures across the two languages. For these grammar tasks, we deliberately selected grammatical forms that were functionally similar in Spanish and English. If participants relied on some kind of grammatical 'bootstrapping' from one language to the other, either in the performance on this task or in their acquisition of the forms in question, we could expect high correlations across the languages by structure. To examine whether the knowledge of specific grammatical forms was related, correlational analyses of scores by type of structure were calculated. There were significant correlations for superlatives ($r = 0.40$, $p < 0.001$) and universal quantifiers ($r = 0.25$, $p = 0.014$), but not for any other structure. Quantifiers are similar in linguistic formation in English and Spanish, in the sense that quantifiers in both languages are pre-nominal (*every N, cada N*). However, this is not the case with superlatives. As mentioned earlier, superlatives in English are formed by inflecting adjectives with the suffix *–est*, whereas in Spanish they are formed by adding a definite article before *más/menos* 'more/less' and the adjective. We speculated above that the bilinguals may have been using their knowledge of English superlatives to answer the superlatives in Spanish in a fashion that was different from the monolingual Spanish speakers. This possibility is potentially supported by the fact that the superlative is one of the only two forms that show a correlation in performance across the two languages.

If the individual structures do not on the whole show correlations in performance across the two languages, the overall high correlation between the overall scores for the two grammar tasks most likely arises through some mechanism other than direct linking between parallel structural types across languages. One possibility is that a person who is good at learning grammatical structure (or performing on a test of the type here) will be good at doing that for both languages. Another possibility, in keeping with proposals in Gathercole *et al.* (in press), is that there are links at a level other than a morphosyntactic one between the two languages – e.g. at an underlying conceptual level or at a metalinguistic or metacognitive level. For example, in order to interpret correctly a declarative sentence such as 'the boy kissed the girl' (i.e. determine whether it is the boy or the girl doing the kissing), one must be able to represent the argument structure and assign thematic roles to the nominal elements of the sentence, regardless of whether it is in English or Spanish. Grammatical knowledge may be related in the bilingual mind in the sense of grammatical meaning rather than grammatical form.

SES effects

Although the participants of this study were all college students or graduates, they came from a mixed socio-economic background as children. It has been observed that low-income (low-SES) children often have less linguistic input from adults (Hoff, 2006) and tend to have lower linguistic skills than their middle class (mid-SES) peers (Hart & Risley, 1995; Hoff, 2003; Lee & Croninger, 1994). As a result, low-SES preschoolers have been shown to have smaller vocabularies, as well as lower levels of the requisite linguistic and cognitive skills needed for learning, and perform more poorly on literacy and academic skills. The varied socioeconomic backgrounds of the participants here when they were growing up allow us to examine whether there are any long-term effects of early experience observable in adult bilingual speakers' grammatical knowledge.

In order to address the issue of SES effects on performance, the bilinguals were divided into SES groups according to the mother's education, the father's education, the mother's profession and the father's profession for each bilingual during his/her childhood. Education was categorized as primary, secondary, university or post-graduate; professions were classified into three levels, 1 for white collar/professional, 3 for blue collar and 2 for intermediate between these. Correlational analyses of these SES indicators with overall performance on the English grammar test and the Spanish grammar test showed a significant correlation (or near-significant correlation) of performance with only the father's profession: for Spanish, $r = -0.355$, $p = 0.002$; for English, $r = -0.216$, $p = 0.059$. This indicates that the higher the father's professional level, the better the performance on the grammar tasks.

The data were re-analyzed to examine more closely the relation of SES, with the father's profession as a proxy for SES, with performance on the grammar tasks. The ANOVAs reveal a main effect of SES on performance for the Spanish grammar task ($F (2, 74) = 7.59$, $p = 0.001$), but not on the English grammar task ($F (2, 74) = 2.28$, $p = 0.109$). Figure 5.4 visually shows bilinguals' performance on English and Spanish by level of SES when the father's profession is taken as a proxy variable. Scheffe's multiple comparisons reveals that for Spanish, there were significant differences in performance between adults whose fathers were white collar workers versus those whose fathers were of an intermediate or blue collar profession, $p = 0.003$, $p = 0.019$, respectively.

It is interesting that, as with the origin home language groups, differential performance by level of SES is observed in Spanish, but not in English. That is, long-term effects of early experience related to SES level can be observed in the bilinguals' performance for the minority language (Spanish), but not the majority language (English) in the community, even in a group of adults that is supposedly homogeneous in terms of educational experience (all of them were college students or graduates).

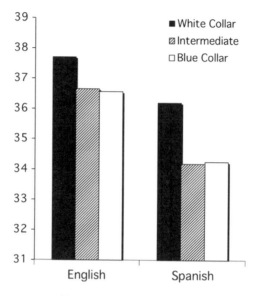

Figure 5.4 Performance on English and Spanish by SES (Father's profession), Bilinguals

Discussion

Bilinguals' and monolinguals' performance on the English grammar task did not differ, not even in the case of L1S-L2E bilinguals, who can be considered to have had the least exposure to English. In Spanish, we found that ESH bilinguals performed less well than L1S-L2E bilinguals, and that OSH and ESH bilinguals performed less well than the L1S-L2E bilinguals and the Spanish monolinguals on SO relative clauses. Furthermore, the bilinguals performed differently from the Spanish monolinguals on some structures, such as superlatives and time conjunctions. These latter effects are likely attributable to the bilinguals' carry-over of English distinctions to Spanish.

When scores on the two tests were compared, overall performance in English and Spanish was highly correlated, but individual parallel structures largely were not. Thus, bilinguals tend to perform equally well in English and Spanish, but the relationship is likely at a cognitive or metalinguistic or metacognitive level. Finally, there was an effect of SES level, as judged by fathers' professions, on bilinguals' performance in Spanish, but not in English.

These results should be interpreted in the context of the sociolinguistic situation in Florida and more generally the United States. Although Spanish is one of the predominant minority languages, English is still the language of communication outside the home and the Hispanic community, and it is also the primary language of education and professional advancement. In the

State of Florida, English is the official language (Article II, Section 9, proposed by Initiative Petition filed with the Secretary of State August 8, 1988; adopted 1988). The bilinguals taking part in the study had spent all or most of their lives in the United States, and had received their education in English. The results of this study suggest that the input they had received in English provided comparable exposure, in the long run, to the grammatical structures, in that their ultimate outcomes were similar to those of the English monolinguals. By the time they were tested (as adults), there was no evidence of any differences that might have manifested had they been tested as children (see Gathercole *et al.*, this volume).

It is worth noting explicitly that these results on the English grammar task show very clearly that being bilingual is not detrimental to the bilinguals' knowledge of English, contrary to often expressed fears in the lay sector.

The story is different for Spanish, for which bilinguals with the greatest exposure to this language (the L1S-L2E bilinguals) performed better than those with the least exposure (the ESH bilinguals). The Spanish input the bilinguals had received appears to provide a more variable experience in terms of quantity and quality than the English input, so that the ultimate outcomes in Spanish remain distinct across the home language types. In the case of Spanish, then, the results of the grammar task highlight the fact that the Spanish the bilinguals develop differs in subtle ways from that of Spanish monolinguals. This asymmetry between majority and minority language has been attested for other language pairs and ages (see Gathercole *et al.*, this volume). It is striking that we find this effect attested even in this highly educated group who might be considered those having optimal opportunities for success in their two languages.

Design of the Assessment Instruments

In closing, a few remarks concerning the design of the test for assessing grammatical proficiency in bilinguals are in order. With regard to designing a measure for grammatical testing, there is the question of whether to use similar grammatical forms, at least in terms of function, or different grammatical forms (see Peña *et al.*, 2013). Using similar forms, the choice followed here, allows comparing performance on items that play comparable functions across languages. Including forms that differ in the two languages – e.g. for the two languages tested here, one could include grammatical gender for Spanish, mass/count for English, null vs. pronominal subjects for Spanish, verbal particles for English, expressions of topic through word order in Spanish, or auxiliary fronting for question formation in English – allows one to examine the extent to which a speaker has acquired the structure of the given particular language.

Whereas the ideal for developing a normed test might be one that includes both types of structures, one could use a test similar to the one presented here to provide norms for development in bilinguals that would give information on both languages in tandem. Although the adults tested here showed an equally high level of proficiency in English, there were differences in their Spanish. And we have successfully employed the comparable tests for Welsh-English bilingual children to differentiate children's abilities from distinct home language groups in development. Those data reveal consistent differences in profiles of development related to level of exposure to the two languages (see Gathercole & Thomas, 2009). A similar set of data for Spanish-English bilingual children will allow us to provide similar profiles for children developing those two languages.

Conclusion

This chapter has addressed the assessment of grammatical knowledge and abilities in bilinguals, focusing on the performance of adult Spanish-English bilinguals (brought up and living in the US) compared to monolinguals. It raises a number of issues concerning the assessment and testing of bilinguals for linguistic abilities, as well as grammatical knowledge.

One of the main issues concerns the interpretation of differential performance in bilinguals and monolinguals. Bilinguals sometimes perform differently from monolinguals, but this is not necessarily because their linguistic knowledge is impaired. The results of our study show clearly that differential language exposure has an effect on performance. It is clear that, if these bilinguals had been tested in only one language, the picture of their language abilities would be incomplete (if tested only in Spanish, their language skills might have been underestimated). The fact that even these highly educated bilingual speakers show subtle differences in their end-state processing of Spanish suggests that we might find similar or even more dramatic effects in other populations of bilinguals (younger, less highly educated, and so forth). Potential differences of this kind support arguments for testing bilinguals in both languages for a more accurate assessment of their linguistic abilities.

Another related issue is the use of monolingual norms when assessing bilingual populations. A bilingual's organization of a language can be different from that of a monolingual, due to cross-linguistic influence. The results of our study suggest that cross-linguistic influence has some effect on performance, highlighting the need to obtain and use bilingual norms (as well as monolingual norms) when assessing bilingual populations.

The fact that bilinguals' performance in each of their languages can be affected by level of exposure has implications for language policy and education. The results of our study indicate that the practice of assessing bilinguals in only one language does not provide an accurate picture of their language abilities. Also, measuring them against monolingual standards or targets needs to be undertaken cautiously and intelligently, because it does not allow for differences in performance due to differential language exposure or cross-linguistic influence. Studies such as the one presented in this chapter provide a better understanding of the factors behind similarities and differences in the performance of bilinguals and monolinguals. Educators, practitioners, and policy makers can draw on studies such as this to make informed decisions about bilingual education, to develop appropriate interventions and strategies, to interpret results on assessments, and to promote good policy and practice with bilinguals.

Acknowledgments

This work is supported in part by ESRC & WAG/HEFCW grant RES-535-30-0061, ESRC grant RES-062-23-0175, and a WAG grant on the Continued Development of Standardised Measures for the Assessment of Welsh, for which we are very grateful. We would like to thank research assistants Garamis Campusano and Jessica Miller for their work recruiting participants and collecting the data, and Florida International University for their support. We are also grateful to Miami Dade College for its help in recruiting participants for this study, particularly to Dr Graciela Anrrich, Professor of ESL/Foreign Languages for her assistance in recruitment and logistics of testing, to Stephen Johnson and Dr Michelle Thomas for their personal support, and to the participants themselves. This research would not have been possible without their collaboration.

References

Bishop, D.V.M. (1979) Comprehension in developmental language disorders. *Developmental Medicine and Child Neurology* 21, 225–238.

Constitution of the State of Florida: As revised in 1968 and subsequently amended - Online document: http://www.leg.state.fl.us/Statutes/index.cfm (Retrieved 01-08-2011)

Cook, V. (ed.) (2003) *Effects of the Second language on the First.* Clevedon: Multilingual Matters.

Crawford, J. (2004) *No Child Left Behind: Misguided approach to school accountability for English language learners.* Washington, DC: National Association for Bilingual Education, Center on Education Policy.

Döpke, S. (2000) Generation of and retraction from cross-linguistically motivated structures in bilingual first language acquisition. *Bilingualism: Language and Cognition* 3(3), 209–226.

Gathercole, V.C.M. (2007) Miami and North Wales, so far and yet so near: Constructivist account of morpho-syntactic development in bilingual children. *International Journal of Bilingual Education and Bilingualism* 10 (3), 224–247.

Gathercole, V.C.M. and Hoff, E. (2007) Input and the acquisition of language: Three questions. In E. Hoff and M. Shatz (eds) *The Handbook of Language Development* (pp. 107–127). NY: Blackwell Publishers.

Gathercole, V.C.M., Laporte, N. and Thomas, E. (2005) Differentiation, carry-over, and the distributed characteristic in bilinguals: structural 'mixing' of the two languages? In J. Cohen, K.T. McAlister, K. Rolstad and J. MacSwan (eds) *Proceedings of the 4th International Symposium on Bilingualism* (pp. 838–851). Somerville, MA: Cascadilla Press.

Gathercole, V.C.M., Pérez-Tattam, R. and Stadthagen-González, H. (in press) Bilingual construction of two systems: To interact or not to interact? In E.M. Thomas and I. Mennen (eds) *Unravelling Bilingualism: A Cross-disciplinary Perspective*. Bristol: Multilingual Matters.

Gathercole, V.C.M. and Thomas, E.M. (2009) Bilingual first-language development: Dominant language takeover, threatened minority language take-up. *Bilingualism: Language and Cognition* 12, 213–237.

Gathercole, V.C.M., Thomas, E.M. and Hughes, E. (2008) Designing a normed receptive vocabulary test for bilingual populations: A model from Welsh. *International Journal of Bilingual Education and Bilingualism* 11 (6), 678–720.

Grosjean, F. (1985) The bilingual as a competent but specific speaker-hearer. *Journal of Multilingual and Multicultural Development* 6, 467–477.

Grosjean, F. (1989) Neurolinguists, Beware! The bilingual is not two monolinguals in one person. *Brain and Language* 36, 3–15.

Grosjean, F. (1998) Studying bilinguals: Methodological and conceptual issues. *Bilingualism: Language and Cognition* 1, 131–149.

Hart, B. and Risley, T.R. (1995) *Meaningful Differences in the Everyday Experience of Young American Children*. Baltimore, MD: Brookes.

Hernandez, A., Bates, E. and Avila, L. (1994) On-line sentence interpretation in Spanish-English bilinguals: What does it mean to be 'in between'? *Applied Psycholinguistics* 15, 417–446.

Hoff, E. (2003) Causes and consequences of SES-related differences in parent-to-child speech. In M.H. Bornstein and R.H. Bradley (eds) *Socioeconomic Status, Parenting, and Child Development* (pp. 147–160). Mahwah, NJ: Erlbaum.

Hoff, E. (2006) How social contexts support and shape language development. *Developmental Review* 26, 55–88.

Kilborn, K. and Ito, T. (1989) Sentence processing strategies in adult bilinguals. In B. MacWhinney and E. Bates (eds) *The Crosslinguistic Study of Sentence Processing* (pp. 257–291). Cambridge: Cambridge University Press.

Kupisch, T. (2007) Determiners in bilingual German–Italian children: What they tell us about the relation between language influence and language dominance. *Bilingualism: Language and Cognition* 10 (1), 57–78.

Lee, L. and Canter, S. (1971) Developmental sentence scoring: A clinical procedure for estimating syntactic development in children's spontaneous speech. *Journal of Speech and Hearing Disorders* 36, 315–340.

Lee, V.E. and Croninger, R.G. (1994) The relative importance of home and school in the development of literacy skills for middle-grade students. *American Journal of Education* 102, 286–329.

Müller, N. and Hulk, A. (2001) Crosslinguistic influence in bilingual language acquisition: Italian and French as recipient languages. *Bilingualism: Language and Cognition* 4, 1–21.

No Child Left Behind Act (2001) – Online document: http://www2.ed.gov/policy/elsec/leg/esea02/index.html (Retrieved 30-09-2011)

Oller, D.K. and Pearson, B.Z. (2002) Assessing the effects of bilingualism: A background. In D.K. Oller and R.E. Eilers (eds) *Language and Literacy in Bilingual Children* (pp. 3–21). Clevedon: Multilingual Matters.

Paradis, J. (2000) Beyond 'One system or two?': Degrees of separation between the languages of French-English bilingual children. In S. Döpke (ed.) *Cross-Linguistic Structures in Simultaneous Bilingualism* (pp. 175–200). Amsterdam: John Benjamins.

Pearson, B.Z. and Fernández, S. (1994) Patterns of interaction in the lexical growth in two languages of bilingual infants and toddlers. *Language Learning* 44, 617–653.

Pearson, B.Z., Fernández, S. and Oller, D.K. (1993) Lexical development in bilingual infants and toddlers: Comparison to monolingual norms. *Language Learning* 43, 93–120.

Peña, E.D., Bedore, L.M. and Fiestas, C. (2013) Development of bilingual semantic norms: Can two be one? In V.C.M. Gathercole (ed.) *Solutions for the Assessment of Bilinguals* (pp. 103–124). Bristol: Multilingual Matters.

Purpura, J.E. (2004) *Assessing Grammar.* Cambridge University Press.

Tomasello, M. (2003) *Constructing a Language: A Usage-based Theory of Language Acquisition.* Harvard University Press.

Toronto, A.S. (1976) Developmental assessment of Spanish grammar. *Journal of Speech and Hearing Disorders* 41, 150–171.

United States Census Bureau (2009) *Selected Social Characteristics* - Online document: http://factfinder.census.gov/ (Retrieved 01-08-2011)

6 Assessment of Bilinguals' Performance in Lexical Tasks Using Reaction Times

Miguel Á. Pérez, Cristina Izura, Hans Stadthagen-González and Javier Marín

In this chapter we describe some ways in which cognitive tasks used in psycholinguistic research can be used to assess the language skills of bilingual speakers. We present a description of the processes involved in picture naming, visual lexical decision and word categorization tasks, and some applications of the tasks for assessing the different aspects of lexical representations. The possibility of knowing the 'mental time' needed by a given participant to process individual words (as measured via response times) might be one of the most important contributions from these tasks. We examine the use of response time measures for assessing the language skills of bilingual speakers. An empirical study recently carried out by our research group provides an illustration of how to examine the acquisition of L2 vocabulary using the tasks and techniques presented in the chapter. The aim of this study was to assess whether the order in which vocabulary is learned affects the 'quality' of the representations formed. Results on accuracy and response times are interpreted with respect to the task-specific demands and in the light of theoretical models.

Introduction

In this chapter we present some ways in which cognitive tasks and techniques can be used to assess the language skills of bilingual speakers. We describe several cognitive tasks commonly used in psycholinguistic research to assess lexical aspects, and we encourage the use of response time to improve bilingual and second language assessment, because it allows greater precision in the detection of subtle differences between subjects or tasks, or across time. Subsequently, we illustrate all with an empirical study,[1] demonstrating how to examine the acquisition of L2 vocabulary using reaction times.

Potential Contributions to Bilingual and Second Language Assessment from Psycholinguistic Research Methodologies

Traditionally, cognitive, linguistic and psycholinguistic research on language acquisition and processing has attracted only, or mainly, the interest of other cognitive, linguistic and psycholinguistic researchers. This may be because it has generally been held that results obtained in laboratory settings cannot be generalized *directly* to what happens in natural contexts, possibly because the tasks used in the laboratory are different from those that any individual engages with while learning or using a language. Although this may to some extent be true, research trends have changed, and it has become increasingly important in scientific research not only to make significant advances in our knowledge of a particular subject but also to find concrete and practical applications and direct them appropriately to ultimately benefit the wider community. As a consequence, much effort is nowadays devoted to bridging the gaps between theory and practice and to making a more explicit impact on policy making, general practice and teaching.

The tools of analysis commonly used in psycholinguistic research are one part of the scientific method that has enormous potential to be adapted in innovative ways to the assessment of second language learning and proficiency. In addition, recent technological advances are providing users with operating mechanisms that are increasingly economical and easier to use. Technological developments (e.g. touch screens) have made commonly used psycholinguistic tasks and techniques affordable and accessible to environments beyond the laboratory (such as for assessing children's language in a school setting).

A wide range of cognitive tasks are used in psycholinguistic research to assess the type of information (e.g. orthographic, phonological and/or semantic) an individual uses and/or needs when processing a word. They are also used to evaluate the nature of morphological, syntactic or semantic analyses individuals engage in during sentence processing.

The linguistic questions that can be examined with these tools range from general, as for example whether an individual knows a word, to more specific enquiries in which the level of phonological, orthographic, or semantic knowledge can be assessed, as well as the time it takes an individual to identify or pronounce a word (as an indicator of how hard it is to access and retrieve the word). These aspects are very interesting in the context of language assessment in general, but are even more important in the context of bilingualism and second language learning because they provide the means to answer complex questions such as whether the bilingual speaker processes words more efficiently and quickly in one language than the other, whether his or her L2 processing is equivalent to that of a monolingual speaker, or what kind of acquired skills a person differentially develops in L2 comprehension as opposed to L2 production.

The possibility of knowing the 'mental time' needed by a given participant to process individual words (as measured via response times) might be one of the most important contributions from these tasks and techniques. We will examine the use of RT measures for assessing the language skills of bilingual speakers, and then illustrate all with an empirical study recently carried out by our research group.

Beyond Accuracy Rate: Response Times as a Richer Measure of Linguistic Performance

Our knowledge about a particular topic or the specific skills we acquire over time has been traditionally measured by developing questionnaires or experiments and then computing responses in such a way that they reflect respondents' knowledge/expertise in a given domain. Questionnaires provide a simple, cheap and effective way to assess knowledge, and they can provide scores for use by evaluators as an 'objective' way of making decisions, e.g. on whether an individual is ready to pass a course, which applicant is the best candidate for a job, or even whether a pattern of responses may be considered pathological. Psychometric theories have been amply developed to determine the best way to design and use questionnaires to collect reliable and valid information from participants' answers (see e.g. Nunnally, 1967; Rasch, 1992).

In cognitive experimental research, the primary behavioural measure to determine the effectiveness in a given task is the accuracy at which individuals respond to a question or stimulus. If the individual answers correctly, for example to name an object, it is assumed that s/he has successfully carried out the cognitive and motor processes to complete the task. If the answer is incorrect, incomplete, or simply missing, it is considered an error, and it is assumed that one or more of the processes involved in the tasks have not been carried out successfully.

Beyond these, however, one prime behavioural measure is response or reaction time (RT). Response time is the interval of time between the onset of a stimulus and the onset of a response. This is usually measured in milliseconds. The time needed to respond to a given item is usually overlooked by common ability tests. However, experimental psychologists have long been using reaction time as one of the most informative measures to determine the nature of the cognitive processes that underlie behaviour. Response times, along with response accuracy and the accuracy/speed trade-off, constitute the metrical basis that current cognitive experimental psychologists use to uncover the nature of mental processes (Meyer *et al.*, 1988; Pollatsek & Rayner, 1998; Posner, 1978).

We can draw inferences from RTs and accuracy combined regarding the mental processes underlying a particular task. These inferences are based on the simple assumption that mental computations (at the functional level) and brain operations (at the neurophysiological level) need time (Donders, 1969; Sternberg, 1969). Complex behaviours demand more processes and need more time than simpler ones. For example, for a simple task in which participants have to press a button when a dot appears on a screen, a single (and short) RT would be expected because the task completion only needs (a) the stimulus detection and (b) the response execution. For a more complex task in which participants are instructed to press '1' if the stimulus is an 'X' and '2' if the stimulus is an 'O', RT is expected to be longer because, besides requiring (a) stimulus detection and (b) response execution, such a task requires (c) discrimination between stimuli and (d) selection of a response.

To gauge processing in complex tasks, two methods involving RTs are common: The *subtractive method* (Donders, 1968) and the *additive factor method* (Sternberg, 1969). Both methods assume that mental processes are sequential in nature (i.e. process B starts as soon as process A finishes). Donders' method involves measuring RT twice, first in a simple task (e.g. press a key when a dot appears on the screen), and then in a subsequent task in which an additional process is needed (e.g. press a key if a dot appears on the screen but do not respond if a star appears on the screen). The difference between the two RTs serves as an estimation of the duration of the additional process embedded in the more complex task (i.e. the discrimination process). This method has received criticisms regarding the assumptions about the independence and sequential timing of processes (McClelland, 1977; see below).

The *additive factor method* (Sternberg, 1969) addresses the problem of the independence of processes (or stages of processing) by distinguishing between 'stages' and 'factors'. Stages are theoretical constructs that represent a *'series of successive processes that operates on an input to produce an output'* (Sternberg, 1969, p. 282). Factors are experimental conditions manipulated by the experimenter. Each factor may influence one or various stages. If two factors affect different stages the contribution to the response time will be additive. If these factors affect at least one common stage the shared contribution to RT will depend on the specific combination of levels of each factor. For example, the time to recognize a word may be affected by lexical frequency (Factor 1) and by the size of the font (Factor 2). If both factors affect separate stages of processing, their effects will be additive: that is, the contribution of the font size (small, big) to word recognition speed will be the same for high frequency as for low frequency words. If there is an interaction between factors, it would then be concluded that font size and word frequency are associated with at least one common (the same) processing stage. In any case, interpreting independence or interactive effects of factors simultaneously manipulated should always be undertaken within the perspective of theoretical models, which propose the number and nature of processing stages for a specific skill.

A particularly interesting point for the assessment of individual differences is exploring when there is an interaction of experimental factors with subject factors. In some experiments it is possible to introduce factors that reflect individual differences, such as *reading level* (e.g. normal vs. dyslexic). When pure experimental factors (lexical frequency, regularity, etc.) interact with subject factors we can infer which processing stages are not working well and may be responsible for any deficit observed. For example, word frequency – a hallmark in lexical access research (Coltheart *et al.*, 1977; Forster, 1976) – predicts a difference in word recognition time by word frequency for normal readers, who recognize high frequency words more quickly than low frequency words. However, the size of this effect is much smaller or is completely absent in surface dyslexics. This is taken as indicating a poor functionality in the access to the orthographic lexicon in the normal reading activity of dyslexics (Castles & Coltheart, 1993; Coltheart *et al.*, 2001).[2]

Although RT is widely used in psycholinguistic experimental research, its employment is nearly absent from standard procedures assessing psycholinguistic abilities. A detailed review of the reasons behind this is beyond the scope of this chapter. However, we believe that an important contributing factor may be the limitations of access to the adequate technological instruments to measure the RT associated with verbal behaviour in standard assessing contexts. Fortunately modern computers provide a good solution to this problem. Current technology makes it relatively easy and inexpensive to measure response times accurately (in milliseconds) across different linguistic tasks and assessment contexts. The only requirement is a computer and an experimental generator program to present the task and to record a participant's responses. Other devices such as a microphone, headphones, a keyboard, gamepad, response box and voice-keys are also used, depending on the nature of the task and the type of response required from participants. The timing of events should be as accurate as possible, and this implies perfect synchronization between stimulus presentation and response registering, and several commercial data collection programs are now available. Some of the most commonly used experimental generator software are DirectRT (Jarvis, 2010a), MediaLab (Jarvis, 2010b), E-Prime (Schneider *et al.*, 2002) and SuperLab (Cedrus, 2011). Freeware options that are at least of equal quality are: Affect (Hermans *et al.*, 2004), DMDX (Forster & Forster, 2003), and Expyriment (Krause & Lindemann, 2011). (See Table 6.1 for information on how to access these programs.) In all cases,

Table 6.1 Software tools for time response collecting

Software	Company	Freeware	Web
DirectRt	Empirisoft	No	http://www.empirisoft.com/directrt.aspx
MediaLab	Empirisoft	No	http://www.empirisoft.com/MediaLab.aspx
E-Prime	PST, Inc.	No	http://www.pstnet.com/eprime.cfm
Superlab	Cedrus	No	http://www.superlab.com/
Affect	See web	Yes	http://fac.ppw.kuleuven.be/clep/affect4/
DMDX	See web	Yes	http://www.u.arizona.edu/~jforster/dmdx.htm
Expyriment	See web	Yes	http://code.google.com/p/expyriment/

learning to use this type of software is not difficult, particularly for the design of standard and simple tasks.[3]

The advantages of using RTs to assess psycholinguistic abilities and verbal behaviour are many. One of the most important is that using the same type of measures (both performance and timing) in research and in applied contexts makes it easier to relate scientific theories and models with applied contexts. Most of the effects found in the laboratory are based on speed of correct responses, not just percentage of correct responses. Incorporating RT measures into language assessment will lead to more adequate explanations of the phenomena of interest. By focusing perhaps too much on behavioural responses such as categorization and classification of pure surface features, we may have been developing explanations that have involved secondary causes rather than primary causes. With the advent of the available tools, more sophisticated measures can now easily be incorporated into applied contexts. These will complement descriptive assessments with assessments linked to explanatory models of language processing, and in the end they will lead to improved measures in psycholinguistic and educational settings.

Another advantage of using RTs in the evaluation of language competence is their high precision. RT measurement allows the detection of subtle differences between subjects, tasks, or across time. RTs can serve as the basis of a new index of difficulty in a psychometric sense. If an individual has to respond to two different words, questions or items in a given test, and he or she answers both correctly, the difficulty of those questions could be explored further by attending to the latency of each response. In a similar vein, if two individuals take the same test and get the same number of correct responses, it would be possible to tell whether the test was equally difficult for them by examining the total time they needed to provide the answers (for some examples, see the discussion below and Figures 6.5 and 6.6, p. 153). Why might one individual be faster than another when responding? Individual differences might arise for various reasons, ranging from the level of ability/automaticity an individual has developed through life (Norman & Shallice, 1986; Posner & Snyder, 1975) to strategies they may have developed, to educational differences, to age, gender, health and the like. Similarly, why do some stimuli need less processing time than others? Processing time depends on a large number of factors varying from the complexity of the task to the characteristics of the stimuli. For example, reading a word aloud depends, among other things, on its frequency, the place in the visual field in which it is situated, the way in which its orthographic form is sounded, its lexical status, etc. Thus, high-frequency words with a predictable pronunciation (e.g. *mint, hint* and *tint)* and presented in the centre or in the right visual field, are recognized more quickly than invented words or low frequency words with unpredictable pronunciation (e.g. *pint)* or items presented in the left visual field (Fiebach *et al.*, 2002).

Finally, another potential approach to the use of RT in language assessment is the possibility of test standardization based on mean-item-RTs. The mean RT of an item can give an estimation of the difficulty of that item for a given population. By finding items that are equated for mean RT, we could bypass problems of translation or, more generally, of linguistic particularities in psychological assessment. For example, if a given word in a reading comprehension test shows different RTs for children born in different parts of the country (or from different socio-economic classes, cultures, etc.), we can suspect that this word is not the same for the different populations. However, if we manage to adapt the item (changing words, syntax and so on) so that the different populations answer it in a very similar time (and accuracy, obviously), we could assume that the two forms of the items have the same psychometrical properties. Using such equivalents could allow one to develop parallel forms of a given test.

Different Cognitive Tasks to Assess Different Aspects of Lexical Processing

Accuracy and response time are usually registered in the most common psycholinguistic tasks used for assessing the representational status of isolated words. Both measures are used to infer how the manipulated factors affect the cognitive processes involved in each task. In the following sections, we present a description of given processes and some applications of the tasks for assessing the different aspects (i.e. orthography, phonology and semantics) of lexical representations.

Lexical decision

The lexical decision task is commonly employed to study the processes involved in word recognition, both in the auditory and visual modality. Individuals are typically asked to decide, as fast as they can, if sequences of sounds they hear or letters they see represent real or invented words.

Participants usually respond by pressing one key if they consider the stimulus to be a word and a different key if they believe it is an invented word.

It is assumed (Young & Ellis, 1995) that to reach the correct decision, one of two mental dictionaries or *lexicons* is accessed. The *auditory* lexical decision forces participants to access the phonological lexicon, whereas the *visual* lexical decision entails access to the orthographic lexicon. However, the processes required to distinguish real from invented words is highly dependent on the nature of the invented words (James, 1975; Richardson, 1976; Rubenstein *et al.*, 1971). When all the invented words presented are formed by consonant strings, conventionally known as *non-words* (e.g. HGB, PTR, NBVG), a mere visual screening will be enough to reach a decision. The individual can easily develop the response strategy of 'every time I see a vowel I report it as a word'. Employing this strategy will result in quick and accurate responses. In contrast, the processes engaged in making a lexical decision response are different when the invented words are orthographically and/or phonologically similar to real words, conventionally known as *pseudowords* (e.g. BURF, MAE, RINT). In these cases determining that a stimulus is a word is assumed to require lexical access (James, 1975; Richardson, 1976).[4]

The lexical decision task is widely used as a relatively valid and reliable measure of word recognition. Higher word recognition competencies are correlated with higher accuracy rates and shorter response times (Balota & Chumbley, 1984). Thus, this task is a useful tool in the assessment of receptive vocabulary knowledge. For example, Meara and Jones (1990) developed the Eurocentres Vocabulary Size Test (EVST) based on a database of 10,000 words that ranged from very low to very high frequency. The EVST consists of a lexical decision task in which participants distinguish 100 words from 50 pseudowords. The words presented represent the range of frequencies comprised in the database. The EVST program makes an estimation of the vocabulary size of the individual based on the number of correct responses observed in relation to the frequency of the words. Another example is DIALANG,[5] which uses the individual's level in a lexical decision task (called 'Placement Test') to adapt the difficulty of subsequent proficiency tests on reading, writing, listening, grammar and vocabulary. Both EVST and DIALANG are based on accuracy rates and not on response times. As we claimed in the former section and we will try to show in the following one, these and other similar assessment tasks can be improved if response times are incorporated. The lexical decision task is easy to implement and can straightforwardly suit the requirements of experts in a range of disciplines (e.g. educators, speech therapists, etc.).

Categorization

In a categorization task, objects or words are commonly displayed visually, and individuals are asked to classify them according to a particular attribute (e.g. 'Is X bigger than a loaf of bread?') or in relation to some pre-defined semantic categories (e.g. living vs non-living items; animals vs fruits and vegetables; natural vs man-made objects). The task is considered to be accessing semantic storage, as the meaning of the referent has to be accessed in order to reach a correct response (Forster, 2004). Participants categorize the stimuli by selecting one of two pre-specified keys.

The categorization task can be considered to be a natural complement to the lexical decision task because, in contrast to the lexical decision task, it ensures that the semantic content of the words (i.e. their meaning) has been accessed. A potential limitation is the development of response strategies that can undermine the interpretation of results. Correct categorization responses can be made via a reflection process based on the two proposed categories, as intended, but also based on one of the categories only (e.g. is this a fruit or not?), or based on a distinctive element of one category (e.g. if the item has legs I say 'animal', otherwise I say 'vegetable'). In these latter cases, the classification is only partially successful because only the items belonging to one category (i.e. fruit) have been processed, or the categorical classification has been completely transformed (from 'animals vs vegetables' to 'legs vs no-legs').

One method that has been designed to circumvent such difficulties is the Go/No-Go procedure. This procedure requires participants to press a key if a pre-specified condition occurs (e.g. if the presented word refers to a living being) and to not respond, that is, to skip the trial, otherwise (i.e. if the presented word does not refer to a living thing). This procedure has some advantages and disadvantages relative to the standard 'yes/no' procedure. In visual lexical decision and categorization tasks, a go/no-go procedure offers faster response times and more accurate responding (Gómez et al., 2007; Perea et al., 2002), especially if the experiments and evaluations involve developing readers (Moret-Tatay & Perea, 2011). The go/no-go technique also requires fewer processing demands, so that it could properly be used in long tasks or in the last tasks of an extensive assessment session.[6]

Semantic categorization tasks examine word knowledge at a deeper level than lexical decision tasks. For example, a student learning a second language might be able to recognize that *earthworm* is a word in a lexical decision task without knowing its meaning–making the response based on the word-like 'feel' (i.e. how word-like a stimulus is) . This makes the semantic categorization task particularly useful in those situations in which word comprehension is important.

Naming

The naming task is widely used in the study of word production (see e.g. La Heij, 2005; Levelt, 1999). During the task individuals are asked to name as quickly as possible objects, colours, words or letters. The nature of the stimuli determines the naming processes.

A simple model that describes well the main stages involved in NAMING PICTURES is that of Marr (1980, 1982). Everything starts with a visual identification process requiring the recognition of the object (i.e. what the object looks like), then the semantic features of the object are activated (i.e. what the object's attributes and properties are), and finally the spoken form corresponding to it from the phonological output lexicon is accessed and retrieved (Levelt *et al.*, 1991). Correct picture naming entails that the individual recognize the stimulus as familiar; know its uses, properties and attributes; and access the phonological form of the picture name.

Object naming applies in multiple contexts. For example, it is a task commonly given to neuropsychological patients (e.g. with The Boston Naming Test by Kaplan *et al.*, 1983) to assess whether the three basic stages mentioned in Marr's model (1980, 1982) are intact. This task can also be used in conjunction with databases of age of word acquisition (e.g. Pérez & Navalón, 2005) to assess whether children's vocabulary develops at an adequate rate.

Successful WORD NAMING or READING WORDS ALOUD depends, in part, on the ability to match familiar printed words with their representations in lexical memory. This ability alone, however, will not ensure the correct pronunciation of all the words a skilled reader might encounter. Vocabulary learning is a never-ending process and as such the reader is likely to encounter novel words throughout life. Naming novel words cannot depend on a matching process as no mental representation has been formed yet. Thus, any word reading account must include a mechanism/s by which familiar and novel words can be read successfully.

The two current leading models of word reading are the dual route and the connectionist model. The dual route model proposes two different mechanisms, one lexical and one non-lexical, to read words aloud (Coltheart *et al.*, 2001). The lexical route has a stored printed and phonological representation for every known word. All familiar words can be read correctly via the lexical pathway irrespective of their regularity (e.g. *kin* is a regular word because the pronunciation of all its letters adheres to the most common pronunciation, /ɪ/, for a written 'i' in the absence of other vowels; conversely, *kind* is irregular, in that the 'i' is pronounced /ai/). The non-lexical route is called the grapheme to phoneme conversion route (GPC) and translates letters (e.g. 'p', 't', 'k'), or groups of letters (e.g. 'ph', 'oo', 'ea'), into their most common sounds. This route can be used to read novel words, pseudowords, and those regular words in the language whose pronunciation can be reliably guessed from their printed forms. According to the dual route model for reading, regular words can be read successfully by either of the two routes, correct reading of irregular words can only occur through the lexical route, and novel words can only be read via the non-lexical route.

The triangle model (Harm & Seidenberg, 2004; Seidenberg & McClelland, 1989), drawing on connectionist theory, proposes a single processing system for reading all known words, irrespective of their regularity, and all unknown novel words. This is achieved by means of a learning mechanism that extracts the statistically more reliable (frequent) spelling-sound relationships in the language.

Naming tasks are designed using experimental generation packages whose software synchronizes stimulus presentation with a trigger that is activated by the first sound produced by the participant. This sound is recorded through a microphone attached to a head set with a voice-key connected to the computer. The recorded responses can then be reviewed, both for accuracy and response time, offline by the evaluator.

Training and Assessment of Foreign Words Learned in a Controlled Setting: Order of Acquisition Effects

The following study provides an illustration of how to examine the acquisition of L2 vocabulary using several of the techniques mentioned above. The aim of this study was not the assessment of the vocabulary that was being learned but whether the order in which vocabulary is learned affects the 'quality' of the representations formed. The training task and the tests used could be applied to any training and assessment program for L2 or bilingual learners.

The *Age/Order of Acquisition* (henceforth OoA) effect on lexical processing is well established (for reviews, see Johnston & Barry, 2006; Juhasz, 2005). The observed effect refers to the fact that, all else being equal, words learned early in life are identified and produced more quickly, and with fewer errors, than words learned later. This effect was first detected in the speed with which English native speakers named a series of pictures (Carroll & White, 1973). The effect has been extensively investigated and observed in a wide variety of languages (e.g. Spanish, Italian, Turkish, German, Greek, etc.). It has been found relevant for many types of tasks (word recognition, word naming, lexical decision, semantic categorization, translation, writing to dictation, etc.), and has been found in distinct populations (bilingual speakers, children, younger and older adults, patients with language difficulties) (Johnston & Barry, 2006; Juhasz, 2005).

At the theoretical level, the OoA effect has important implications for the way of conceiving the adult lexicon, as this effect associates the representational status of words with the time that those words were incorporated into the lexicon. Most models of lexical recognition, comprehension and production include factors that have to do with lexical frequency, length, syllable structure, etc., but they do not include a factor having to do with the timing of lexical learning. So it is a major challenge to implement the effect of OoA into these models.

OoA implications have been less developed at the practical level than at the theoretical level, but we can highlight a study and some potentially promising lines. In one study, Forbes-McKay *et al.* (2005) showed that the age of acquisition of words produced in a semantic fluency task can reliably differentiate normal from pathological age-related cognitive decline. Other studies indicate that the OoA effect has other potential, but challenging, applications. For example, Izura and Ellis (2004) observed in a series of experiments using translation tasks in bilinguals that the OoA effect is specific to the L1 or L2. That is, early-acquired words in L1 (e.g. *bruja*, the Spanish word for 'witch') may show an advantage in processing time with respect to other later-acquired words in L1, but the translations into the L2, if the word is late-acquired in the given language (e.g. *witch*), will show slower processing times than other earlier-acquired words in the L2. Izura and Ellis concluded that OoA may affect lexical processing and access to semantic representations, but not necessarily those semantic representations themselves. Bilingual assessments may be able to take this result into account and develop tasks and tests that control for OoA of the assessed words both in L1 and L2.

Other challenging applications of the OoA effect are directly related to the experiment that we present here. OoA could be taken into account to tune an L2 training programme in order to optimize learning. For example, one could include those words that are usually more difficult to learn at the beginning of training, and leave the 'easiest' words for the latest training stages.

An important question is why or how the OoA effect arises. Two alternative accounts are currently under debate: the semantic hypothesis and the mapping hypothesis. The semantic hypothesis (Brysbaert *et al.*, 2000) suggests that as a consequence of cumulative learning (over time) the concepts of early acquired words develop more semantic connections and, as a consequence, are more firmly embedded in the semantic memory. The mapping hypothesis (Ellis & Lambon-Ralph, 2000) proposes, instead, that OoA effects emerge as a consequence of the loss of plasticity: A neural system or network modifies itself to learn early or first information to an optimal level. As a consequence of maximising optimal learning at the beginning, when the system needs to later learn new information, the network cannot be optimized to the same level, creating a disadvantage for the material learned later.

Before presenting our study, it is worth mentioning up front that there are a number of questions regarding the OoA effect that are still under debate. One is whether the OoA effect is independent from the many other factors with which it correlates, such as word frequency or concreteness (i.e. early acquired words like *bread* tend to be also short, frequent and concrete, Gilhooly & Logie, 1980). Some authors, as a result, consider OoA to be a mediator factor that somehow encapsulates many other factors such as frequency, length and concreteness (Bonin *et al.*, 2004). Other authors have suggested that there is a confounding between OoA and *cumulative frequency*, that is, the total number of times a word is encountered in an individual's lifetime (e.g. Lewis *et al.*, 2001). Still others have argued that the *frequency trajectory,* that is, the distribution of the word frequency over a lifetime, should be used as the genuine measure of age-limited learning effects (Zevin & Seidenberg, 2002).

Another controversy surrounding the OoA effect is the methodology used for collecting the OoA values (i.e. the OoA measurement). The OoA scores used when designing experiments are usually extracted from adults' estimations of the age at which they think they learned a given word (e.g. Gilhooly & Logie, 1980). Although a high level of inaccuracy can be suspected in relation to this way of measuring OoA, the estimations have shown acceptable validity levels, with high correlations between ratings and more objective OoA measures that have been calculated from oral production in children (e.g. Morrison *et al.*, 1997; Pérez & Navalón, 2005).

Study

The present study aimed at assessing the unique contribution of the OoA effect when processing words. In order to control for all intercorrelated factors, the experiment was designed in such way that a group of Spanish native speakers learned a series of foreign words in Welsh under laboratory conditions. Words were introduced into training at different points in time (i.e. early and late) in the course of two weeks, within a highly controlled training paradigm that ensured that all the words were presented the same number of times (i.e. had the same frequency), had the same length, and were equally concrete. It was hypothesized that the observation of an OoA effect within this experimental context would imply that OoA is not an amalgamation of a series of characteristics (e.g. word frequency, letter length, level of concreteness) but an independent source of variance.

Under OoA accounts, the mapping hypothesis predicts age or order of acquisition effects under any situation in which material is learned in a cumulative and interleaved manner (i.e. as in the case of the present experiment). In contrast, the semantic hypothesis predicts that the foreign words (e.g. *buwch* 'cow') would inherit the OoA characteristics of the first-language translation equivalents (in this case, Spanish *vaca*), as the meanings of the words are thought to be learned only once, when learned with the L1, and to be shared between the two languages. Thus, the mapping hypothesis predicts an order of acquisition effect, whereas the semantic hypothesis does not.

Method

The experiment used real Welsh words that were unknown to the Spanish participants at the start of the experiment. The words were shown as second language words to be acquired as part of a vocabulary learning task. Learning occurred in nine sessions spaced over two weeks, one session per day for nine consecutive working days. A set of 'early' words was included into training from the onset, whereas the introduction of 'late' words was delayed until after the participants had spent two days learning the early items. Early items continued to be presented, whereas the later ones were trained. That is, training was cumulative and interleaved. The impact of this training programme on object naming, lexical decision and semantic categorization accuracy and speed of performance was assessed, at short-, medium- and long-term after the end of training.

Participants

Twenty-four undergraduate students from the University of Murcia in Spain (7 males and 17 females) took part in this experiment in exchange for some extra academic credits, and for remuneration in accordance with the number of tests completed. All were native Spanish speakers who had English as a second language (at secondary education level) and were not familiar with Welsh or any other non-native language. They had a mean age of 21;7 years (range 18–41) and did not have any visual or auditory impairments.

Materials

The stimuli consisted of 28 black and white pictures of objects (Pérez & Navalón, 2003) and their Welsh names. All the words referred to familiar concepts for participants (e.g. 'swan', 'tree', 'ear', 'boat'; see Appendix 1). Fourteen of these referred to natural objects and 14 to man-made objects. The object names did not involve any distinctively Welsh phonemes. Object names that were inter-language cognates (i.e. sharing the meaning and form across the two languages) were avoided. The objects and their Welsh names were divided into two sets of 14 each (named as A and B in Appendix 1). The sets were matched on letter and phoneme length, bigram frequency, number of orthographic neighbours, objective OoA of the Spanish translation, word frequency and familiarity of the Spanish translation (Pérez & Navalón, 2003; 2005) (see Appendix 1).

In addition, ratings for the orthographic similarity between the words in Welsh and their translations into Spanish along with picture naming times in Spanish were also collected from other groups of participants. For the former, 21 participants were shown Welsh words and their translations into Spanish and were asked to rate how similar the two members of each pair of words were, on a scale from 1 (not alike at all) to 7 (almost the same). For the latter, 11 participants were asked to name the pictures in Spanish, and accuracy and response times were collected for each item. The word sets used in the experiment were matched on these factors (i.e. orthographic similarity and picture naming performance in Spanish) as well (see Appendix 1).

Conditions were counterbalanced across participants in such a way that one set was presented as the early set to half of the participants and as the late one to the rest, and the other set was presented in the reverse order.

Four lists of 28 pseudowords were created for the lexical decision tasks by changing one letter from each of the Welsh words learned. The pseudowords were therefore similar to the new words being learned during training (see Appendix 2)

Procedure

The experiment comprised a series of training and test sessions.

Training sessions:

Participants followed a training programme of nine sessions over a period of two weeks (see Figure 6.1), during which they were taught, both in oral and written form, 28 Welsh words divided into two sets (A and B) of 14 words each. Early and late sets were presented eight times each in seven training sessions in such a way that the frequency trajectory, the number of sessions, and the sessions' characteristics were exactly the same for both conditions (early and late). Late items were introduced for the first time in training session 3. By the end of the last training session, session 9, every item had been experienced 56 times.

During the training, participants were encouraged to memorize the associations between the pictures and the words in their spoken and written forms. An E-Prime 2 (Schneider et al., 2002) routine controlled the stimulus presentation and response collection. All sessions were carried out in a soundproof booth.

The procedure for presenting pictures and words was as follows: Training sessions 1 and 2 (early set only): An object picture appeared on a computer screen for five seconds, with its Welsh name written below it in lower case. At the same time, the spoken name was presented through headphones in a female voice (a native speaker). Participants were asked to associate the written and spoken Welsh word to the picture, which represented the real meaning. They were also asked to repeat aloud the word within the time allotted. This was done six times for each picture and its corresponding name. After that, participants saw the pictures again for 10 seconds along with

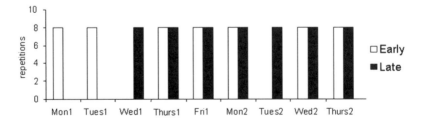

Figure 6.1 Training programme

their spoken and written names. However, on this occasion participants did not have to repeat the word aloud. Instead they were asked to copy the words down on a sheet of paper. This was done twice for each picture and object name. Spoken responses from the repetition task were recorded and reviewed offline by the experimenters, as were the written responses. Training sessions 3 and 7 (late set only): The second set of 14 object-names (late set) was introduced in session 3 for the first time. In sessions 3 and 7, the late words were presented following the same procedure and number of times as in sessions 1 and 2 for the early word set.

Training sessions 4, 5, 6, 8 and 9 (early and late sets): Items from the early and late sets were presented together and in a random order. Each item was presented in the same fashion and number of times as was described above for the early and late sets.

Acquisition tests: On Wednesday and Friday of the first week of training, two acquisition tests were carried out to assess learning. It is important to note that despite this assessment, the training programme went on in week 2 as described above. Participants were asked to produce in their own time the spoken and written names of the early pictures in the first acquisition test, and the names of the late pictures in the second acquisition test. Accuracy of verbal and written responses was later checked by the experimenter.

Main test sessions: There were four testing sessions in which RTs and accuracy for object naming, visual lexical decision, and semantic categorization of written words were collected. These took place 1, 6, 13 and 41 days after the last training session. Participants were encouraged not to rehearse or practice recall of the learned words between testing sessions.

Visual lexical decision task: Participants were shown the 28 trained words interleaved randomly with 28 pseudowords. Right-handed participants were asked to press the 'M' key, if they considered the item on the screen to be a word and the 'Z' key if they considered it to be a pseudoword. Left-handed participants used the 'Z' key for words and the 'M' key for pseudowords. Each trial started with a central fixation cross for 200 ms., followed by a blank screen for 250 ms. A word or pseudoword was then presented until a response was registered or until a timeout of 2700 ms. occurred. Finally, an inter-trial blank screen appeared for 1000 ms. Presentation of items was randomized across participants and sessions. Stimuli were presented and accuracy and RTs of responses were recorded using E-Prime (Schneider *et al.*, 2002).

Picture naming task: Each trial began with a fixation cross appearing in the centre of the screen for 350 ms., followed by a blank screen for 200 ms. Then a picture from one of the trained items was presented for 3000 ms. or until a response was registered, during which time participants were encouraged to produce the Welsh name for the item as quickly and as accurately as possible. The screen then went blank for 500 ms. before the next trial began. Presentation of items was randomized. Presentation of pictures and responses and RT recordings were controlled by using DMDX (Forster & Forster, 2003). This software allows the recording of verbal responses online through a microphone connected to the computer's soundboard. Responses were later coded as correct or incorrect offline by the experimenter. In order to identify trials in which hesitations or strong exhalations had accidentally activated the voice key, all sound files were inspected visually using Checkvocal (Protopapas, 2007).

Semantic categorization task: The 28 experimental words referred to 14 natural objects and 14 man-made objects. Each trial in the categorization task began with a fixation cross for 200 ms. The screen then went blank for 250 ms., and then one of the learned words was presented for 2500 ms. or until a response was made. Finally, an inter-trial blank screen appeared for 1000 ms. A 'go/no-go' technique was used. Half the participants were asked to press a key if the word was the name of a natural object and not to respond if the name referred to a man-made object. The remaining participants pressed the key if the word denoted the name of a man-made object and made no response if the word was the name of a natural object. E-Prime was again used for item presentation and response recording (Schneider *et al.*, 2002).

Results

Results from the acquisition tests conducted during training showed high learning rates: 79% accuracy on early-trained words in session 3, just after two training sessions, and 82% on late-trained words in session 5, after two training sessions on the late words. Analysis of errors showed that many of them were approximations to the target words (see Figure 6.2).

Picture naming

First, accuracy of responses was examined. Errors were analyzed using Wilcoxon matched pairs, signed ranks tests to compare the number of errors made to early and late items at each test. No OoA effects were found (see top of Table 6.2, Picture Naming).

Analyses of RTs for naming were carried out on correct responses longer than 300 ms. and for times lower than 3 standard deviations above the mean for each participant and testing time (using these criteria, 1.7% of trials were considered to be outliers and were removed from analyses). Mean RTs by participants were subjected to a 2×4 ANOVA with OoA (early, late) and tests (day 1, 6, 13, 41) as within-participants factors. The main effect of tests

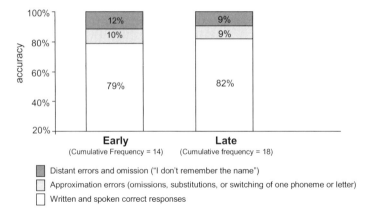

Figure 6.2 Results of acquisition tests

approached significance, $F(3,63) = 2.441$, mse $= 17651.6$, $p = 0.073$, $\eta_p^2 = 0.10$, with the first test taking less time than the rest (919 ms. for test 1; 974 ms. for test 2; 944 ms. for test 3; and 990 ms. for test 4). The mean RT to early and late introduced words was exactly the same (957 ms.), so no significant OoA effects were found, $F(1,21) < 1$. The interaction between tests and OoA was not significant $F(3,63) < 1$. An additional ANOVA ($2 \times 2 \times 4$) was carried out adding order of presentation of sets (henceforth, just 'set') as a between-

Table 6.2 Response error rates (%) by task, OoA and test

	Test1 (1 day)	Test2 (6 days)	Test3 (13 days)	Test4 (41 days)	Overall
Picture naming					
Early items	7.4	7.7	7.1	11.3	8.4
Late items	5.7	6.8	6.5	11.3	7.6
All items	6.5	7.3	6.8	11.3	8.0
Lexical decision					
Early items	4.2	2.7	3.0	5.1	3.7
Late items	4.5	3.0	4.8	2.4	3.6
All items	4.3	2.8	3.9	3.7	3.7
Pseudowords	6.3	9.8	7.8	10.1	8.7
Categorization					
Early items	3.6	4.8	2.4	6.5	4.3
Late items	3.6	1.8	2.4	1.8	2.4
All items	3.6	3.3	2.4	4.2	3.3

subjects factor. No main effect or interactions involving set were found, and no alteration to the pattern of results obtained for the other factors was observed.

Lexical decision

Only responses to the Welsh words were analyzed. First, errors to the newly-learned words were analyzed using Wilcoxon matched pairs, signed ranks tests to compare the number of errors made to early and late items at each test. No OoA effects were found (see Table 6.2, Lexical Decision section).

RTs shorter than 300 ms. and longer than 3 standard deviations above the mean for each participant were considered outliers and removed from further analysis (1.1%). The patterns of RTs across sessions are shown in Figure 6.3. Mean RTs by participants were subjected to a 2×4 ANOVA with OoA and tests as factors. The main effect of tests was not significant, $F(3,63) < 1$. The main effect of OoA was marginally significant, $F(1,21) = 4.307$, MSe = 5702.5, $p = 0.050$, $\eta_p^2 = 0.17$, with faster overall RTs to early words (832 ms.) than to late words (856 ms.). The interaction between tests and OoA was not significant, $F(3,63) = 4.307$, MSe = 2348.5, $p = 0.092$, $\eta_p^2 = 0.09$. A further ANOVA ($2 \times 2 \times 4$) was carried out with set as an additional factor. No main effect or interactions involving set were found, and no alteration to the pattern of results obtained for the other factors was observed, except that the effect of OoA appeared clearly significant, $F(1,20) = 5.822$, MSe = 4217.9, $p = 0.026$, $\eta_p^2 = 0.63$.

Word categorization

Errors were analyzed using Wilcoxon matched pairs, signed ranks tests to compare the number of errors made to early and late items at each test. No significant differences between early and late sets were found, except in test 4, where, paradoxically, late items were responded with fewer errors (1.8%) than early items (6.5%), $Z = -2.326$, $p = 0.020$ (see Table 6.2).

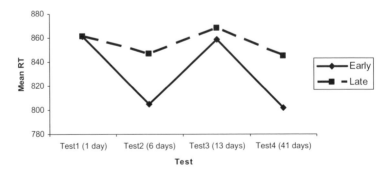

Figure 6.3 OoA effects in lexical decision

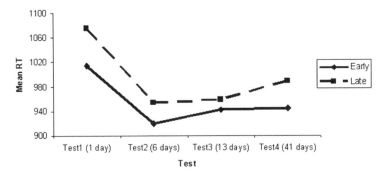

Figure 6.4 OoA effects in categorization

Mean times of correct 'go' responses were calculated. Analyses of RTs were carried out on correct 'go'-responses longer than 300 ms. and less than 3 standard deviations above the mean for each participant and testing time (1% removed). Participant and item mean RTs were subjected to a $2 \times 4 \times 2$ ANOVA with OoA, tests and response category (natural objects or manmade objects) as factors. The main effect of tests was highly significant $F(3,63) = 6.362$, MSe $= 16871.4$, $p = 0.001$ $\eta_p^2 = 0.23$. The main effect of OoA was also significant, $F(1,21) = 4.927$, MSe $= 13943.6$, $p = .038$, $\eta_p^2 = 0.19$. As is shown in Figure 6.4 RTs declined across tests, with a clear advantage for early over late items at every test. Overall, RTs were faster for the early words (955 ms.) than for the late words (994 ms.). The main effect of response category was not significant, and none of the interactions were significant, $F(1,21) < 1$.

An additional ANOVA $(2 \times 2 \times 2 \times 4)$ was carried out adding set as a factor. No main effect of set was found, and no alteration to the pattern of results obtained for the other factors was observed.

Discussion

The following conclusions can be drawn from our data. According to the processes that take place in the picture naming task, an individual that responds correctly to the task necessarily had to activate the semantic features associated with the object and then the phonological form to pronounce the name. The high percentage of correct answers displayed in this task (92%) and its maintenance over time reflects success in the training. This is not a trivial result, considering the number of foreign words to be learned, the number of training sessions conducted, and the fact that the associations between pictures (meanings) and phonological forms were completely novel to participants. Additionally, the Welsh words used in the experiment had very few phonological and orthographic neighbours with respect to Spanish words as a whole, so the phonotactic structures of the learned words were not analogous to words in Spanish. On the other hand, the mean RT in this task was 957 ms., which may suggest that the spoken production of the Welsh words, although taking more time than when individuals produce words in their native tongue (approximately 600 ms.; Levelt *et al.*, 1999), shows some command of these words by the participants. Finally, taken all together we can infer that participants built complete and stable phonological representations during the training programme, and these remained for several weeks even without explicit training.

On the basis of the characteristics and the obtained results from the visual lexical decision task (participants showed an overall accuracy rate of over 96%), it seems clear that participants can discriminate correctly the trained items as words from other very similar forms that are not words.[7] That means that they generated visual (orthographical) representations of words associated with their corresponding meanings. The high accuracy observed in this task demonstrates the training programme effectiveness in the acquisition of written forms of words, too (see Table 6.2). The average response time for the Welsh words was 843 ms. Although it is not surprising that this time is higher than those normally found in the same task with L1 words (approximately 500 ms. in visual lexical decision, Forster (1976)), it is noteworthy that the mean time is lower than that found for the same items in the picture naming task. This matches the findings on the comparison between the two tasks when performed in L1, because, as is widely established (see Levelt *et al.*, 1999), accomplishing a picture naming task needs more processes (and may be more complex, too) than are needed for completing a lexical decision task. On the other hand, response times obtained in the visual lexical decision task served to reveal differences in processing between early and late learned words, even though no differences were observed for accuracy (see Table 6.2 and Figure 6.3).

Finally, the word categorization task allowed us to test whether participants established connections between the visual forms of words and their meanings. Although we used simple and concrete concepts, the stimuli were useful for ruling out the possibility that participants had used some kind of strategy based on a non-linguistic visual memory to perform the lexical decision task. In order for participants to be able to say whether the word on the screen referred to a natural or artificial object, they had to access the meaning of the word. The high percentage of correct answers given by the participants in this task (96.7%) implies that the training programme served for the establishment of lexical-semantic associations. The average response time shown by the participants to complete the task was 975 ms. If this time is compared with that obtained in the lexical decision task we see that the former is somewhat higher, which also fits with the predictions coming from the evidence found in L1. Word categorization tasks require additional processes on top of those required for performing a lexical decision task. In a categorization task, in addition to lexical access, individuals need to activate semantic associations with the given word. In this case individuals have to activate enough semantic information to decide if the referenced object was natural or man-made. Response times obtained in the categorization task also allowed us to observe that participants were statistically significantly slower in the first test (1045 ms.) than in the later tests (937 ms. in the second, 950 ms. in the third test, and 967 ms. in the fourth). This result could seem counter-intuitive, because one would expect that the more time passes without explicit training or rehearsal, the greater the increment in response times will be. Although this issue requires more investigation, one possible explanation could come from the fact that the first main test was the first time that participants were aware of the possibility of grouping the trained words as referring to natural or man-made things. Therefore, in the first test participants may have showed a slower response than in subsequent tests because the classification as natural or artificial objects entailed a novel criterion. This could have slowed down the decision-making processes, whereas in the rest of the tests the classification was made from a known criterion, which could then be carried out more quickly. On the other hand, one might hypothesize that the learning of semantic information needs more time for organization and consolidation, so effects are better when medium or long-term memory are involved. In any case, we also have to consider that we do not really know what participants did after training despite the fact that they were encouraged not to rehearse the learned words on their own between testing sessions.

Relevance and validity of the present results

Following Izura and colleagues (2011), we tried to simulate real-life OoA effects in the laboratory by manipulating the moment at which new words entered into training in a task involving learning foreign language vocabulary. For accuracy of performance, there was no difference by OoA on any of the tests. But for reaction times, we found significant effects of OoA for the lexical decision and semantic categorization tasks, but no effect of OoA in picture naming. The evidence of a null effect of OoA in picture naming does not match the results observed previously in Izura et al. However, the significant OoA effects observed for the lexical decision and semantic categorization tasks cannot be explained in terms of the frequency of exposure to different items, because these were matched for the early and late sets. Those OoA effects were sustained over a 41-day period after the end of training.

The present effects are consistent with current theories of OoA, particularly the mapping hypothesis (Ellis & Lambon-Ralph, 2000; Lambon-Ralph

& Ehsan, 2006). This hypothesis claims that memory systems progressively lose plasticity and become entrenched as a result of cumulative learning. Learning of new (late) material will be easier if the new representations can exploit network structure created in previous learnings, but it will be more difficult if the new representations require the large-scale formation of new interconnections, or associations that are at variance with those acquired earlier. In our experiment, the OoAs of words in Spanish were matched between sets, and all of the words referred to familiar meanings, so the learning that caused the OoA effects would be related to new orthographical and phonological information (Welsh words) and/or their novel connections to the pre-established meanings.

Assessing the phonological, orthographical and semantic representational status of the newly learned words

The acquisition tests completed two days after training showed a high learning rate (80%) for the association between the form and the meaning of the word. Half of the incorrect answers were approximation errors (i.e. omissions, additions or transpositions of one phoneme or one letter), which indicates some degree of acquisition for those words as well. The tests consisted of two tasks, a spoken and a written picture naming task. According to the reference model, to successfully perform both tasks, an individual first has to recognize the picture, then to access its semantic features and finally to activate the phonological or orthographical representations.

Results from the main tests administered after training also showed a high rate of learning, which continued for several weeks without the existence of any more rehearsal. Accuracy and reaction times were measured from the picture naming, lexical decision and categorization tasks. Comparisons were made between two groups of words, early and late, whose differences in response time made it clear that their OoAs play a role in learning and accessing them.

Response times could also be used in other ways, for example, to analyze and classify participants by their response speeds or to examine the learning evolution during or after training. Moreover, as we have noted, response times enable better discrimination between participants or items, or between different moments of assessment, especially when participants show very good performance on the task (see Yap *et al.*, 2012). In Figures 6.5 and 6.6 we can see an example of these possible analyses. Figure 6.5 shows mean recognition times for the four fastest (*arian, godre, coes* and *afal*) and four slowest words (*ceiriosen, cawrfil, cwningen* and *oriadur*) in the visual lexical decision task. It is important to note that these items were correctly recognized by over 95% of participants in each test (23 out of 24 participants). In the absence of differences in accuracy rate, response times can be used as a

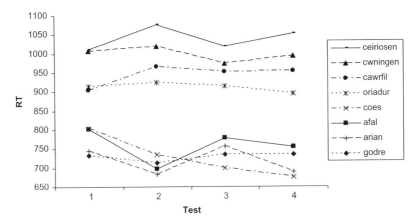

Figure 6.5 The fastest and slowest recognized items with high accuracy rates in visual lexical decision

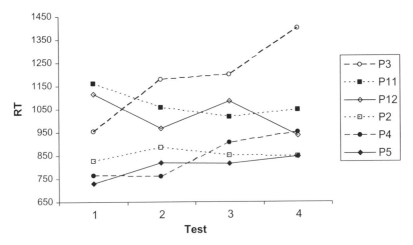

Figure 6.6 Mean response times of some participants with high accuracy rates in visual lexical decision

difficulty index in learning and recalling. In this case, differences owing to word length should be further examined, because it seems that the longer words were recognized more slowly than the shorter ones. In Figure 6.6 we show the differences in mean response times between some participants with accuracy rates over 95% (0 or 1 error out 28 items) in each test of the lexical decision task. As can be see, P3, P11 and P12 were slightly slower than P2, P4 and P5, although some variations in speed can be noted for some participants across the tests.

Final Statement: Response Time, Cognitive Tasks and Language Assessment

In this chapter we have shown some possibilities of how measuring the 'mental time' needed to process isolated words can improve language assessment. Measuring response times, which nowadays is relatively easy to perform in any context, complements descriptive assessments with assessments linked to models of language processing. Moreover, using response times in the assessment of language competence allows a higher precision in the detection of subtle differences between subjects or tasks, or across time (for example, looking for differences in response times between participants who otherwise show equivalently good performance on a task). Finally, we have proposed that mean response times of items could also be used to improve the psychometric standardization of language assessment tests.

As RT measures become incorporated into such assessments, we need to remember that response times always have to be interpreted with respect to the task-specific demands and in the light of theoretical models. We have presented three of the most common tasks used in psycholinguistic research on lexical recognition (visual lexical decision and semantic categorization) and production (naming). Through several examples and an experiment of word training, we have shown how to interpret differences in response times between experimental factors or individuals with respect to the processing stages in word recognition and production, and have suggested possible implications for language assessment.

Notes

(1) This research was supported by the Spanish Ministry of Science and Innovation (PSI2008-03481/PSIC).
(2) There is some debate regarding the exact timing of processing and its manifestation in reaction times. McClelland (1977), for example, criticised the assumption of a sequential status of processing stages. He suggested that the computation of processes may start without the need for previous processes to be finished. This means that processing stages may start to build their outputs as soon as some information from the preceding stages is available. (This mechanism of processing is known as the cascade model.) This implies in practice that an overlap in time between different processing stages may obscure the establishment of direct correspondences between changes in response times and the processing composition. It is by now generally assumed that there is not a simple method to establish the contributions that specific functional components make towards a behaviour and its temporal structure, although models differ in the posited processing stages or in the suggested temporal and functional relations between assumed components (see for example the 2-route vs. triangle model debate in reading). Only through the accumulation of empirical and convergent evidence, including behavioural measures, cerebral imaging and neurological patients, will we ultimately be able to choose in favour of one possibility over others.

(3) It is important to note that RT measures cannot be applied to all tasks. First, RT measures require some degree of speed in the responses. In some cases this kind of response is simply not possible because of particularities of the task. In these cases RT collection is not possible, generally when the task reaches a high degree of cognitive complexity. In those cases in which it is possible to ask for participants to give their responses as quickly as possible (and with no error), there is a trade-off between speed and accuracy. In addition, it is known that some populations, such as very small children, may have problems in understanding speed/accuracy instructions, and that cultural factors may have an important effect in RT (Geisinger, 2003).

(4) The lexical decision task has been criticized because it involves a decision-making response (word versus pseudoword), an extra linguistic process that can add noise to the response times.

(5) DIALANG is a language diagnosis system developed by many European higher education institutions. It reports one's level of skill in terms of the Common European Framework (CEF) for language learning (http://www.lancs.ac.uk/researchenterprise/dialang/about.htm)

(6) It is important to note that following this procedure only half of the information is recorded, at least in response times, because in the 'no-go' condition responses are not recorded.

(7) Contrasts between words and pseudowords were done in order to observe a lexicality effect. Wilcoxon non-parametrical analyses were carried out on error means by participants. They showed significant lower error rates for words than for pseudowords in all the tests (see table 2), $Z = -2.048$, $p = 0.041$ in test 1, $Z = -2.187$, $p = 0.029$ in test 2, $Z = -2.453$, $p = 0.014$ in test 3, and $Z = -2.280$, $p = 0.023$ in test 4. However, one should have in mind that those differences can partially or totally be attributable to hand dominance (see procedure).

References

Balota, D.A. and Chumbley, J.I. (1984) Are lexical decisions a good measure of lexical access? The role of word frequency in the neglected decision stage. *Journal of Experimental Psychology: Human Perception and Performance* 10, 340–357. http://dx.doi.org/10.1037/0096-1523.10.3.340

Brysbaert, M., Van Wijnendaele, I. and De Deyne, S. (2000) Age-of-acquisition of words is a significant variable in semantic tasks. *Acta Psychologica* 104, 215–226.

Castles, A. and Coltheart, M. (1993) Varieties of developmental dyslexia. *Cognition* 47, 149–180.

Cedrus Corpotration (2011) *SuperLab* (Version 4.5.) [Computer Software]. San Pedro, CA, USA.

Coltheart, M., Davelaar, E., Jonasson, T. and Besner, D. (1977) Access to the internal lexicon. In S. Dornic (ed.) *Attention and Performance VI*. New York: Academic Press.

Coltheart, M., Rastle, K., Perry, C., Langdon, R. and Ziegler, J. (2001) DRC: A dual route cascaded model of visual word recognition and reading aloud. *Psychological Review* 108, 204–256.

Davies, W.D. and Kaplan, T.I. (1998) Native speaker vs. L2 learner grammaticality judgments. *Applied Linguistics* 19, 183–203.

Donders, F.C. (1868/1969) On the speed of mental processes. Translation by W.G. Koster in W.G. Koster (ed.) *Attention and Performance II* (pp. 412–431). Amsterdam: North-Holland Publishing Co.

Ellis, A.W. and Young, A.W. (1988) *Human Cognitive Neuropsychology*. Hove, UK: Psychology Press.

Ellis, R. (1991) Grammaticality judgments and second language acquisition. *Studies in Second Language Acquisition* 13, 161–86.

Ferrand, L. and New, B. (2003) Semantic and associative priming in the mental lexicon. In P. Bonin (ed.) *Mental Lexicon: Some Words to Talk about Words* (pp. 25–43). New York, NY: Nova Science Publisher.

Fiebach, C.J., Friederici, A.D., Müller, K. and von Cramon, D.Y. (2002) fMRI evidence for dual routes to the mental lexicon in visual word recognition. *Journal of Cognitive Neuroscience* 14, 11–23.

Forster, K.I. (1976) Accessing the mental lexicon. In E.C.T. Walker and R.J. Wales (eds) *New Approaches to Language Mechanisms*. Amsterdam: North-Holland.

Forster, K.I. (2004) Category size effects revisited: Frequency and masked priming effects in semantic categorization. *Brain and Language* 90, 276–286. http://dx.doi.org/10.1016/S0093-934X(03)00440-1

Forster, K.I. and Forster, J.C. (2003) DMDX: A windows display program with millisecond accuracy. *Behavior Research Methods, Instruments, & Computers* 35, 116–124.

Frenck-Mestre, C. (2005) Eye-movement recording as a tool for studying syntactic processing in a second language: a review of methodologies and experimental findings. *Second Language Research* 21, 175–198.

Geisinger, K.F. (2003) Testing and assessment in cross-cultural psychology. In J.R. Graham and J.A. Naglieri (eds) *Handbook of Psychology. Vol 10: Assessment Psychology*. Hoboken, NJ: John Wiley & Sons

Gómez, P., Ratcliff, R. and Perea, M. (2007) A model of the go/no-go task. *Journal of Experimental Psychology: General* 136, 389–413.

Harm, M.W. and Seidenberg, M.S. (2004) Computing the meanings of words in reading: Cooperative division of labor between visual and phonological processes. *Psychological Review* 111, 662–720,

Hermans, D., Clarysse, J., Baeyens, F. and Spruyt, A. (2005) *Affect* (Version 4.0) [Computer software; retrieved from http://www.psy.kuleuven.ac.be/leerpsy/affect4]. University of Leuven, Belgium.

Izura, C. and Ellis, A.W. (2002) Age of acquisition effects in word recognition and production in first and second languages. *Psicológica* 23, 245–281.

Izura, C. and Ellis, A.W. (2004) Age of acquisition effects in translation judgement tasks. *Journal of Memory and Language* 50, 165–181.

Izura, C., Pérez, M.A., Agallou, E., Wright, V.C., Marín, J., Stadthagen-González, H. and Ellis, A.W. (2011) Age/order of acquisition effects and the cumulative learning of foreign words: A word training study. *Journal of Memory and Language* 64, 32–58.

Jarvis, B.G. (2010a) *DirectRT* (Version 2010) [Computer Software]. New York, NY: Empirisoft Corporation.

Jarvis, B.G. (2010b) *MediaLab* (Version 2010) [Computer Software]. New York, NY: Empirisoft Corporation.

Kaplan, E., Goodglass, H. and Weintraub, S. (1983) *The Boston Naming Test*. Philadelphia: Lea and Febiger.

Krause, F. and Lindemann, O. (2011) *Expyriment* (Version 0.3.2) [Computer Software; Retrieved from http://code.google.com/p/experiment/]. Donders Institute for Brain, Cognition and Behaviour, Radboud University, Nijmegen, The Netherlands

Kroll, J.F. and De Groot, A.M.B. (eds) (2005) *Handbook of Bilingualism: Psycholinguistic Approaches*. New York: Oxford University Press.

La Heij, W. (2005) Monolingual and bilingual lexical access in speech production: Issues and models. In J.F. Kroll amd A.M.B. de Groot (eds) *Handbook of Bilingualism: Psycholinguistic Approaches* (pp. 289–307). New York: Oxford University Press.

Levelt, W.J.M. (1999) Models of word production. *Trends in Cognitive Sciences* 3, 223–232.

Levelt, W.J.M., Roelofs, A. and Meyer, A.S. (1999) A theory of lexical access in speech production. *Behavioural and Brain Sciences* 22, 1–75.

Levelt, W.J.M., Schriefers, H., Vorberg, D., Meyer, A.S., Pechmann, T. and Havinga, J. (1991) The time course of lexical access in speech production: A study of picture naming. *Psychological Review* 98, 122–142. http://dx.doi.org/10.1037/0033-295X.98.1.122

Luce, R.D. (1986) *Response Times: Their Role in Inferring Elementary Mental Organization.* New York: Oxford University Press.

McClelland, J.L. (1979) On the time relations of mental processes: An examination of systems of processes in cascade. *Psychological Review* 86, 287–330.

Meyer, D.E., Osman, A.M., Irwin, D.E. and Yantis, S. (1988) Modern mental chronometry. *Biological Psychology* 26, 3–67.

Moret-Tatay, C. and Perea, M. (2011) Is the go/no-go lexical decision task preferable to the yes/no task with developing readers? *Journal of Experimental Child Psychology* 110, 125–132.

Norman, D.A. and Shallice, T. (1986) Attention and action: Willed and automatic control of behavior. In R.J. Davidson, G.E. Schwartz and D. Shapiro (eds) *Consciousness and Self-regulation: Advances in Research and Theory* (pp. 1–18). New York: Plenum Press.

Nunnally J.C. (1967) *Psychometric Theory.* New York: McGraw-Hill.

Patterson, K.E. and Shewell, C. (1987) Speak and spell: Dissociations and word class effects. In M. Coltheart, G. Sartori and R. Job (eds) *The Cognitive Neuropsychology of Language* (pp. 273–294). London: Erlbaum.

Perea, M., Rosa, E. and Gómez, C. (2002) Is the go/no-go lexical decision task an alternative to the yes/no lexical decision task? *Memory and Cognition* 30, 34–45.

Pérez, M.A. and Navalón, C. (2003) Normas españolas de 290 nuevos dibujos: Acuerdo en la denominación, concordancia de la imagen, familiaridad, complejidad visual y variabilidad de la imagen. *Psicológica* 24, 215–241.

Pérez, M.A. and Navalón, C. (2005) Objective-AoA norms for 175 names in Spanish: Relationships with other psycholinguistic variables, estimated-AoA, and data from other languages. *European Journal of Cognitive Psychology* 17, 179–206.

Pollatsek, A. and Rayner, K. (1998) Behavioral experimentation. In W. Bechtel and G. Graham (eds) *A Companion to Cognitive Science.* Malden, MA: Blackwell.

Posner, M.I. (1978) *Chronometric Explorations of Mind.* Hillsdale, NJ: Lawrence Erlbaum.

Posner, M.I. and Snyder, C. (1975) Facilitation and inhibition in the processing of signals. In P.M.A. Rabbit and S. Dornis (eds) *Attention and Performance.* New York: Academic Press.

Protopapas, A. (2007) CheckVocal: A program to facilitate checking the accuracy and response time of vocal responses from DMDX. *Behaviour Research Methods* 39, 859–862.

Rasch, G. (1992) *Probabilistic Models for Some Intelligence and Attainment Tests.* Chicago: The University of Chicago Press.

Schneider, W., Eschman, A. and Zuccolotto, A. (2002) *E-Prime User's Guide.* Pittsburgh: Psychology Software Tools, Inc.

Sebastián, N., Cuetos, F., Martí, M.A. and Carreiras, M.F. (2000) *LEXESP: Léxico informatizado del español.* [CD-ROM] Barcelona: Edicions de la Universitat de Barcelona.

Seidenberg, M.S. and McClelland, J.L. (1989) A distributed, developmental model of word recognition and naming. *Psychological Review* 96, 523–568

Sternberg, S. (1969) The discovery of processing stages: Extensions of Donders' method. In W.G. Koster (ed.) *Attention and Performance II* (pp. 276–315). Amsterdam: North-Holland.

Yap, M.J., Balota, D.A., Sibley, D.E. and Ratcliff, R. (2012) Individual differences in visual word recognition: Insights from the English Lexicon Project. *Journal of Experimental Psychology: Human Perception and Performance* 38, 53–79.

Appendix 1. Stimuli and their features

Welsh Words	English	Spanish	Category	N	Bi-to	Bi-ty	L	Pho	Freq.	AoA	FA-pic	FA-word	Simil. WLS-SPA	Na-time (SPA)
Set A														
alarch	swan	cisne	Natural	0	322	29	6	4	3.21	93	1.96	5.42	1.30	770
arian	money	dinero	Man-made	0	116	23	5	5	206.96	72	4.47	6.71	1.62	753
brechdan	sandwich	sandwich	Man-made	0	279	39	8	7	0.00	114	3.27		1.38	656
cawrfil	elephant	elefante	Natural	0	266	40	7	7	7.32	30	1.43	5.81	1.38	740
ceiriosen	cherry	cereza	Natural	0	73	21	9	9	0.89	114	3.06		3.38	805
clust	ear	oreja	Natural	0	197	8	5	5	21.96	102	4.59	6.46	1.29	601
crib	comb	peine	Man-made	3	98	6	4	4	5.00	36	4.51	6.55	1.38	673
esgid	shoe	zapato	Man-made	0	306	6	5	5	13.04	36	4.75	6.4	1.24	641
godre	skirt	falda	Man-made	1	1349	15	5	5	21.96	82	3.75	6.29	1.33	741
gwiwer	squirrel	ardilla	Natural	0	213	9	6	6	8.04	72	1.53	5.75	1.40	719
magnel	cannon	cañón	Man-made	0	364	38	6	6	11.96	93		4.41	1.48	901
moronen	carrot	zanahoria	Natural	0	664	67	7	7	2.32	43	3.33	5.56	1.33	718
troed	foot	pie	Natural	0	280	15	5	5	132.68	36	4.71	6.44	1.29	758
utgorn	trumpet	trompeta	Man-made	0	58	9	6	6	3.04	72	1.53	4.69	1.38	762
			MEAN	0.3	327.6	23.2	6.0	5.8	31.3	71.1	3.1	5.9	1.5	731
			SD	0.8	331.8	17.6	1.4	1.4	60.9	30.2	1.5	0.7	0.5	74.8
Set B														
afal	apple	manzana	Natural	3	168	6	4	4	11.07	36	4.33	6.5	1.33	687
agoriad	key	llave	Man-made	0	284	43	7	7	22.86	36	4.65	6.71	1.14	754
breinlen	diploma	diploma	Man-made	0	131	30	8	8	2.14	136	3.00		1.52	787

Welsh	English	Spanish	Type	N	Bi-to	Bi-ty	L	Pho	Freq	AoA	FA-pic	FA-word	Simil	Na-time
coeden	tree	árbol	Natural	0	427	32	6	6	35.00	30	4.06	6.67	1.55	705
coes	leg	pierna	Natural	0	2008	10	4	4	24.64	72	4.65	6.41	1.33	849
cwch	boat	barco	Man-made	0	0	0	4	3	47.68	30	2.10	5.33	1.48	686
cwningen	rabbit	conejo	Natural	0	65	17	8	8	6.61	36	2.31	6.02	1.90	700
edau	thread	hilo	Man-made	1	107	3	4	4	27.68	49	3.25	6.61	1.86	898
gafr	goat	cabra	Natural	2	66	7	4	4	11.25	136	1.65	5.94	2.95	953
gwasgod	vest	chaleco	Man-made	0	32	4	7	7	13.39	102	3.76	6.15	1.43	744
mefusen	strawberry	fresa	Natural	0	420	20	7	7	2.86	49	3.37	6.66	2.05	712
mwgwd	mask	antifaz	Man-made	0	223	3	5	5	1.25	126	2.21		1.38	760
oriadur	watch	reloj	Man-made	0	239	28	7	7	50.71	36	4.41	6.76	2.38	671
trawswch	mustache	bigote	Natural	0	119	28	8	7	22.86	114	2.38	5.61	1.29	685
MEAN				0.4	306.5	16.5	5.9	5.8	20.0	70.6	3.3	6.3	1.7	756
SD				0.9	507.3	13.6	1.7	1.7	16.1	42.5	1.0	0.5	0.5	87.0
π score from τ-test (set A vs. set B)				0.67	0.90	0.27	0.90	1.00	0.51	0.97	0.99	0.12	0.39	0.42

Key: N = number of orthographic neighbours in Spanish.
Bi-to = bigram mean frequency (token) in Spanish.
Bi-ty = bigram mean frequency (type) in Spanish.
L = length in letters.
Pho = length in phonemes.
Freq = lexical frequency (per million) in Spanish.
AoA = age of acquisition in Spanish (in months).
FA-pic = picture familiarity rating.
FA-word = word familiarity rating (subjective lexical frequency).
Simil WLS-SPA = Welsh-Spanish similarity rating.
Na-time = naming times in Spanish.
Databases sources: Sebastián, Cuetos, Martí y Carreiras (2000); Pérez & Navalón (2003, 2005).

Appendix 2. Pseudowords used in each test

Set	Welsh	English	Pseudowords Test 1	Pseudowords Test 2	Pseudowords Test 3	Pseudowords Test 4
A	alarch	swan	alaroh	alarct	atarch	alasch
A	arian	money	anian	aruar	arien	ariar
A	brechdan	sandwich	brechden	blechdan	brecndan	brechban
A	cawrfil	elephant	cawrful	caurfil	cawnfil	cawrvil
A	ceiriosen	cherry	ceiruosen	ceiriacen	ceirioson	ceoriosen
A	clust	ear	crust	clost	clunt	clusf
A	crib	comb	crub	crit	clib	creb
A	esgid	shoe	esged	esgib	engid	esdid
A	godre	skirt	gadre	gogre	godle	godra
A	gwiwer	squirrel	gwider	gwiuer	gwiwes	guiwer
A	magnel	cannon	macnel	magmel	magnil	mognel
A	moronen	carrot	moronin	meronen	morwnen	morohen
A	troed	foot	thoed	traed	troid	troad
A	utgorn	trumpet	utgorm	ulgorn	utdorn	utgosn
B	afal	apple	abal	alal	aful	afat
B	agoriad	key	agoniad	agoried	aboriad	agariad
B	breinlen	diploma	breislen	breinten	breinlwn	bleinlen
B	coeden	tree	coedem	caeden	coeben	coedun
B	coes	leg	cois	coer	cues	coas
B	cwch	sailboat	cuch	cwsh	cwnh	cwct
B	cwningen	rabbit	cwnengen	cwnirgen	cwninben	coningen
B	edau	thread	ebau	edeu	edou	edaw
B	gafr	goat	gafn	gofr	gatr	gavr
B	gwasgod	vest	gwasdod	gwasgud	guasgod	gwangod
B	mefusen	strawberry	metusen	mefuren	mefusin	mafusen
B	mwgwd	mask	mwgwg	mugwd	mwbwd	mwgud
B	oriadur	watch	oriodar	oriabur	oriador	oniadur
B	trawswch	moustache	trawsich	trawswcn	thawswch	trawcwch

7 Assessment and Instruction in Multilingual Classrooms

Rebecca Burns

This chapter addresses the issue of how a (monolingual) teacher can accomplish the assessment and instruction of multilingual and limited L2 proficient students in her classroom. When tests and materials are not available in students' L1, the teacher has available a range of strategies to fill the gaps until the child gains competence in the L2. The creation of multilingual materials is made possible by the wide availability of free digital resources on the internet that are being created by the world's multilingual users. Reasons why teachers might want to assess students using multilingual materials are presented along with guiding principles for their use.

Students and teachers in classrooms around the world are experiencing demands for greater academic achievement to meet national and international standards while at the same time the language differences and disconnects between teachers and students are increasing. Teachers are expected to assess student performance and chart student progress with tools that are standardized for a single language of instruction. Without assessment tools that show students' abilities while they transition to the language of instruction, years of student achievement go unaccounted for. This chapter presents means that teachers can use for informal classroom assessments and to begin instruction for students in any language.

Students follow many different paths to come to a classroom in which they do not understand the language of instruction. The current and the historical migrations of families across political and linguistic borders are increasingly changing the language diversity of schools around the world (Agirdag, 2009). Students who are new learners of the language of instruction in school are likely to have teachers who are monolingual or who are multilingual themselves but may not speak the languages of their students. The students' task of learning both new subject area content and the new language of instruction is made all the more challenging when there is no common language between students and their teachers. Even though standardized assessment tests come in only one language, teachers need access to the multilingual resources of their students for many reasons: to welcome students and their families to the school and the classroom environment, to support students' comprehension of the new language and the new subject matter, and to inform classroom instruction with assessments of students' background literacy and subject area expertise.

Just as the demographics of classrooms are changing around the world, the internet is changing the way teachers and students access information and share resources. Teachers can now access on the web high quality lesson plans designed by experts in standards-based instruction in mathematics, science, language arts, and more. Instructional YouTube videos are increasingly used in classroom settings to free the teacher to focus on individual and small group practice and review. The internet revolution is also multilingual in nature. People around the world are creating digital content in their native languages and making it accessible to the everyday internet user. In countries where internet access is limited, mobile technology such as cell phones is creating text, audio and video avenues of multilingual communication and connection for communities around the world (Cordier, 2011).

This chapter presents basic examples of how multilingual language resources might be used by teachers to create informal assessments and instructional opportunities in their classrooms. The goal of this chapter is to support language awareness for classroom teachers and to promote practitioners' confidence in using assessments in unfamiliar languages for specific, strategic classroom applications. Underlying the goal for this chapter are two important notes:

(1) the suggestions presented for creating multilingual assessment and instructional materials are limited in nature;
(2) the suggestions presented do not represent a substitute for a fully bilingual education experience.

Exploring Assessment Resources for a Multilingual World

There are many reasons why a classroom teacher might want to make the effort to create assessments and instructional materials using the language resources of her students, and they all point toward enhanced learning outcomes. Students and their families may feel more welcome in schools that display greetings and useful information in their familiar languages. Aleman *et al.* (2009) describe the common characteristics of award-winning schools in California: schools with outstanding success rates in producing high academic achievement for every demographic group of students, including populations of English learners of 30% or higher. Surrounding the academic climate in each of the award-winning schools they reviewed was a palpable culture of appreciation of diversity. Appreciation of the diverse languages and cultures of the students and their families was heard and seen throughout these schools at assemblies, in classroom activities, on bulletin boards and on posters in prominent places. Danzak (2011a, 2011b) and Danzak and Wilkinson (2005) report on the importance of a positive bilingual identity in the academic success of Hispanic students and in their social-emotional well-being. English learners with positive bilingual identities were able to deflect the negative effects of language prejudice they experienced in school, were able to participate in high praise classroom events, and were able to create the necessary opportunities to develop highly proficient academic language.

Using home language assessments in classroom teaching also supports acquisition of the target second language and can support students' transfer of cognitive knowledge to the academic demands of the classroom. In their national review of academic achievement of language minority students throughout the US, Thomas and Collier (2002) found that students with 4 or more years of schooling in their primary language (either in the home country or in the host country) achieved academically high levels in English, even when low socioeconomic status would have predicted lower performances. They go on to report that 'Immigrants with interrupted schooling in [the] home country achieved significantly below grade level when provided instruction only in English' (p. 6).

In spite of the strong evidence of positive outcomes for multilingual students who use their home language skills as part of their academic development, using multilingual assessment and instructional materials in schools has typically been thought of as not feasible. For example, the state of Florida has been under a court-ordered Consent Decree since 1990 which requires all public school districts to meet requirements for the identification, assessment, instruction and program monitoring of English learners (LULAC *et al.*, 1990). Each Florida school district must publish their enumerated plan for providing services to students learning English. One of the questions that all districts must answer is whether or not procedures have been developed and implemented to assess ELLs in their native language. Of the 67 school districts in Florida, only 16 answered the question as YES in 2009. Of these 16, only four described a procedure for a language other than Spanish (http://www.fldoe.org/aala/deelp.asp), yet the Florida State Department of Education cites over 220 different native languages for its student population of English learners (http://www.fldoe.org/aala/pdf/1011-ELLsNativeLang.pdf).

It is the position taken in this chapter that indifference to multilingual students' home languages is costly and can no longer be excused as 'unfeasible'. The digital revolution in the global context has brought the languages of the world into data bases, audio files, texts, videos and interactive experiences that are shared at no cost and can be accessed with logical search procedures. In a state such as Florida, which requires all elementary grade teachers to have extensive training in teaching English for speakers of other languages (ESOL), it is imperative that teacher candidates learn to create multilingual assessment and instructional materials for classroom applications. The use of such materials can have positive effects for both the candidates and their students when these materials are introduced during classroom activities. This chapter will recommend a number of free language tools that can be used successfully. Our experience is that even student teachers who are monolingual English speakers and who have had few opportunities to travel internationally or to be immersed in a foreign language environment quickly gain confidence and enthusiasm as the usefulness of multilingual assessment is experienced first-hand.

Getting Started

One of the first ways that a teacher can show support for the languages of her students is to create a multilingual, print-rich environment. Teachers can create customized, multilingual labels for the classroom environment, multilingual word lists of key vocabulary, or multilingual messages to students and parents. Coehlo (2006) provides many suggestions for 'making space' for more than one language in the classroom and in the larger school setting. Coehlo encourages teachers to enlist students, parents and other community speakers of the classroom languages to assist in the creation of multilingual materials, and this is certainly the best way to cultivate a shared interest in such projects.

Teachers can create a home language 'ABC' book with their students who are learning English. The teacher and the student engage in choosing words from the student's language that feature each letter or sound of the English alphabet, write the words in the home language with an English translation and draw pictures to illustrate the meaning of the word. Figure 7.1 illustrates an alphabet poster for an English learner who speaks Spanish at home. The student has a school product that can be shared at home containing new vocabulary in English that is anchored in knowledge of the home language and the picture references. The student and the teacher have learned together that some letters in English are not represented in the student's home language ('w' is not used in Spanish words), that the same letter can sound very different in the two languages (e.g. the trilled 'r' for *rana* ('frog') in Spanish is different from the 'r' in English words). Conscious knowledge of differences and similarities in the use of the alphabet in each of the languages of the classroom is beneficial for both students and their teachers.

However, there are often times when the teacher may not have collaborative help and may wish to prepare multilingual assessments for

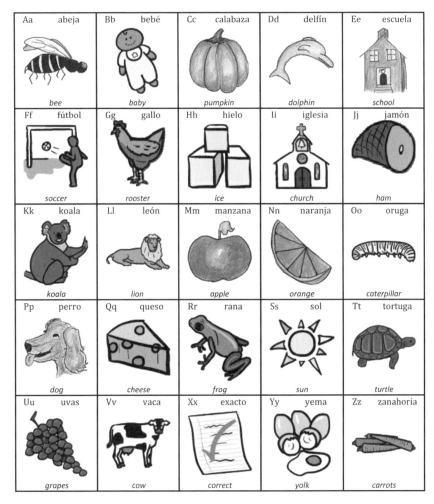

Figure 7.1 ABC book
Source: Images downloaded from UVic Humanities Computing and Media Centre and Half-Baked Software, http://hcmc.uvic.ca/clipart/

strategic instructional purposes. Genesee *et al.* (2013) point out that reading for bilinguals is essentially different from reading for monolinguals because, for one thing, bilingual readers have resources in their additional language(s) for constructing meaning and for checking comprehension. Genesee *et al.* provide evidence for the successful use of home language reading experiences to scaffold early reading instruction and to scaffold later, more complex reading for content-area learning. Teachers will want to create these advantages for their students, and they can create these possibilities with multilingual materials selected for instructional purposes.

Free, Multilingual Online Translators

Creating translated versions of basic classroom assessments and activity materials is now possible through the use of free online translation programs. The number of free online language translators is rapidly increasing and quality is rapidly improving. The popular search engine Google offers a free online translation program that includes over 64 languages, including Haitian Creole, which is the second largest non-English language in south Florida (after Spanish). Google Translate (http://translate.google.com) includes a function that provides synonyms or alternate translations for each item. Another useful online translator is imTranslator (http://imtranslator.com), which features text-to-speech functions for over 50 languages (not including Haitian Creole) and an automatic back-translation function.

Back translation refers to the practice of checking the accuracy of a translation by putting the translated material into the program and requesting translation back into the original language. For instance, if a teacher were translating a test question such as, 'Which of the following processes is responsible for changing liquid water into water vapor?' into Haitian Creole, the translation yields a slightly different form of the question when it is translated back into English: 'Which process is responsible for changing liquid water into water vapor?' The back translation provides a basic check that the intended meaning has been preserved, and it also provides a means for identifying unnecessary words or phrases (such as 'of the following') in the design of test questions. Teachers might use translation software to create multilingual lists of key vocabulary items. A preschool teacher introducing the song, 'Head, shoulders, knees and toes' in a multilingual pre-Kindergarten classroom might want to be prepared to say those four main body parts in the languages of the students in the class, e.g. English, Spanish, Haitian Creole and Ukrainian. Entering each of the four English words into Google Translator and checking back translations, the teacher may come up with the list in Table 7.1.

Translation opens opportunities to understand some important aspects of the languages that students are speaking at home. For example, the expression *dedos de los pies* looks like a very long expression for the simple

Table 7.1 Multilingual vocabulary list

English	Spanish	Haitian Creole	*Ukrainian
head	cabeza	tèt	guolovka
shoulders	hombros, espaldas	zepòl	plyechi
knees	rodillas	jenou	kolinakh
toes	dedos de los pies	zòtèy	palʲtziv

*Ukrainian is shown in a roman script

concept of 'toes'. Back-translating just the Spanish word *dedos* yields *fingers*, so *dedos de los pies* refers to the 'fingers of the feet'. The teacher has discovered an important aspect of naming body parts in Spanish and can better help students learn the English words *fingers, toes* and *digits*. Google Translate offered two different Spanish words for *shoulders*. The teacher can ask students to indicate which word is the better fit, and the teacher can verify the choice with other Spanish speakers as well as continue to research the use of the two words using online searches. When translating *head* into Ukrainian, Google Translate offers up a long list of Ukrainian synonyms for *head*. The synonym list allows us to see that choosing the word described as *head, cap* is more likely to be a body part reference than the words described as *head, leader, manager*. Again, the accuracy of the translation must be verified by the speakers of the language, young and old alike. Teachers may feel challenged by this level of uncertainty in using translation; being unsure of one's self is not usually thought of as a characteristic of an effective teacher. However, being curious to know the outcome of several working hypotheses about words and their meanings is an energetic, positive characteristic of good teachers.

Google Translate produces Ukrainian text written in the Cyrillic alphabet. The teacher will want to convert the Ukrainian words into the Latin alphabet in order to be able to attempt to pronounce the word to the student. The free, online Ukrainian to Latin Converter from MyLanguages.org (http://mylanguages.org) was used for the list shown in Table 7.1. Making attempts to pronounce useful words in the students' familiar languages can help young children activate their prior knowledge as they participate in new language activities. If the teacher points to the referent and makes an effort to pronounce the foreign word, decoding as one would in English, the student typically recognizes the attempted word and provides the correct pronunciation.

By preparing a classroom activity and assessment with multilingual materials, the teacher is prepared to activate the students' multilingual awareness during the activity. This is likely to make the activity more meaningful for all the students as they participate in learning new words together and get to know more of the inner worlds of their classmates. But the multilingual materials prepared for classroom activities also support academic learning objectives. The teacher can use students' familiar vocabulary to assess letter naming and sound-letter correspondences. For older students, translations of vocabulary lists and sentences can be useful for keeping newcomers on schedule with the academic content. A teacher candidate reported that his third grade student, a new arrival from Poland, was very confused by the lesson identifying subjects and predicates. The next day the candidate presented the pupil with the same sentences translated into Polish and the student then understood the concept and could accurately identify the subject-predicate components of any number of Polish sentences.

Language Learning Websites for Vocabulary and Pronunciation

Teachers can access expertly translated materials by using resources provided on language learning websites. Byki Express (http://www.byki.com) features free language learning software in over 70 languages. The programs are formatted as multi-media sets of flash cards for learning vocabulary and short sentences or phrases. Each flash card shows the word in the target language and in English along with a full color picture or photograph and an audio pronunciation of the target word. A turtle icon adjusts the speed of the audio pronunciation. Learners select the word set and interact with each card through a progression of looking, listening and keyboard responses. The program provides right/wrong feedback and keeps a record of scores and progress. The presentation is visually appealing, the photographs are attractive, the cards turn as they show front and back, and the user's score visibly increases with each right answer. Figures 7.2 to 7.4 show a sequence of cards when the Haitian Creole word *zwazo* is entered.

Because Byki uses English translations for its instructions on all word lists, teachers in English-speaking education settings can use Byki Express

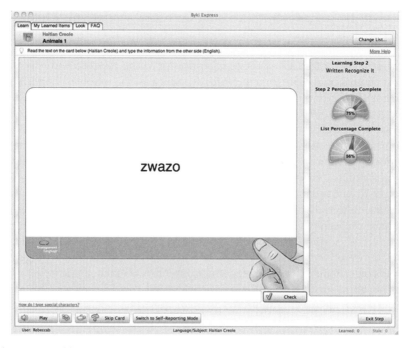

Figure 7.2 Byki 'zwazo'

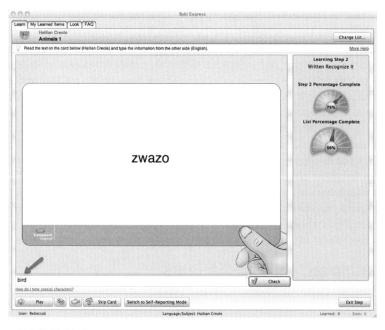

Figure 7.3 Byki 'bird'

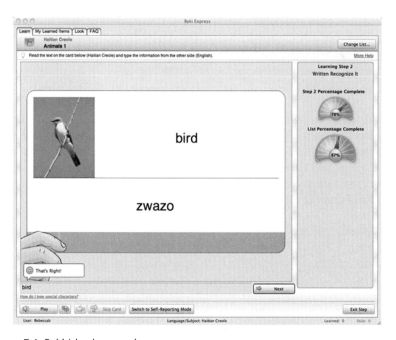

Figure 7.4 Byki 'check answer'

with their English learners whose home languages are represented in the Byki word lists. The lists are searchable by theme and by language. Available lists include basic semantic sets such as animals, foods, numbers, colors; pragmatic sets such as greetings, safety, questions; and grammatical sets such as verbs, connectors and tenses. The Byki word lists can be accessed online, or the lists and the program can be downloaded for offline use. Teachers can print the bilingual word lists as stand-alone documents. Figure 7.5 illustrates Haitian Creole-English word lists generated by Byki.

The Byki List Central community features word lists (all free) contributed by community members. Teachers can sign up to share their lists and to communicate special requests for subject-specific content word lists in the home languages of their classrooms. One might prepare words in languages A and B for, say, Florida endangered species, and upload those to the website, to be used by others.

Multilingual, Multimedia Texts

Multilingual students will benefit from reading extended texts in their familiar languages to support their understanding of classroom learning objectives. As Genesee *et al.* point out (2013), multilingual students are still learning the classroom language, and their reading of grade level texts in the new language will not be as proficient as that of their monolingual peers. Teachers can provide multilingual reading materials and assessments to support and evaluate the content knowledge students must acquire. As multilingual students gain proficiency in the language of the classroom, they will also gain proficiency in using the cognitive strategies effectively used by proficient bilinguals, such as *translanguaging*.

> The term translanguaging, as originally proposed by Cen Williams (1994), refers to Welsh-English bilingual pedagogical practices where students hear or read a lesson, a passage in a book or a section of work in one language and develop their work in another, for example by discussion, writing a passage, completing a work sheet, conducting an experiment... (Hornberger & Link, 2012: 268)

One obvious source for subject-specific content in multiple languages is Wikipedia. Official Wikipedias have been created in 285 languages (http://meta.wikimedia.org/wiki/list_of_Wikipedias). If one wishes to teach a science lesson about plant respiration, or cellular respiration, for example, and wanted to collect definitions and explanations of this concept in the languages of her students, she could put the search terms into Wikipedia (in English, for this example). An article appears which resembles an undergraduate college text. It has eight sections, several chemical formulae and

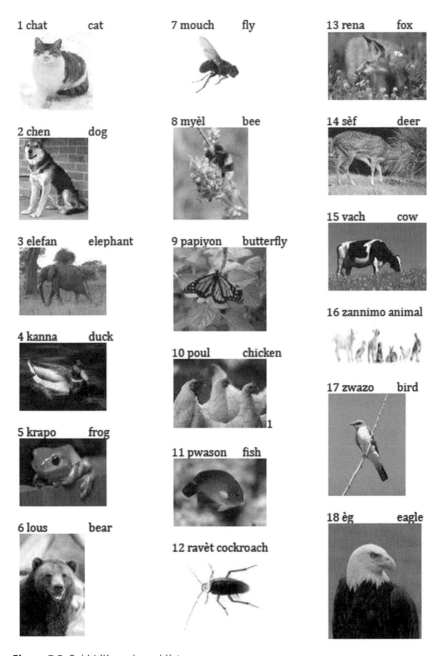

Figure 7.5 Byki bilingual word list

three diagrams. It contains more detail than young students can use, so one can look to the list of languages on the left margin of the article page to see if this article is available in Simple English. It is, in addition to 41 other languages. Clicking on Simple English, one finds 'cellular respiration' discussed with one simplified formula that is also written out in word form, one diagram and five main sections that are very short. On the left side of this page are also listed the languages for which this article may be accessed. The articles do not follow the format of the Simple English article, and each article is very different. The Krèyol ayisyen (Haitian Creole) page has only a definition; the Spanish page is lengthy and resembles a college text. Teachers can determine what assistance, if any, these home language resources are, and can work from the Simple English form to translate key phrases, whole paragraphs and tests.

Multilingual resources for children's literature are a very important consideration in multilingual classrooms of children learning to read. The International Children's Digital Library (http://www.childrenslibrary.org) is a collection of scanned copies of thousands of children's books in over 60 languages. The library is searchable and is also available as an app for portable smart electronic devices. The library website itself is currently available in 16 languages. Mamalisa (http://www.mamalisa.com) is a free website featuring children's song lyrics in over 120 languages. Audio versions of many of the songs are available. The site also hosts international collections of rhymes, poems, recipes and holiday materials. Cultural understanding and language are the overarching themes.

One of the most important uses teachers need to make of multilingual materials is to assess the literacy skills their students have developed in their home languages. For older students, a writing sample in the home language can give some indication of confidence and proficiency, and an informal assessment might be offered by an educated native speaker. But it is more challenging to determine what word recognition skills and story-listening experiences young children have had in their home languages. By providing relevant text material in the home language (packaging of foods typically used in the child's home is a good resource for familiar print), teachers can assess students' responses to and comprehension of print. Classroom teachers are encouraged to assess and monitor their students' reading in all of their languages as it is an important means of determining whether or not a student has a reading difficulty. Reading difficulties generally affect the reader in each of her languages, a very different experience from being limited in reading only the new language (Genesee *et al.*, 2013).

To test students' listening comprehension in the home language, and to support continued development of complex listening, teachers may collect recordings of texts that will serve the instructional purposes of the class. Audio recordings of books may be available, and native speakers may volunteer to create needed materials for one's classroom. YouTube (http://youtube.com)

can be searched for appropriate video materials in the target languages that may be used with only the audio to check students' listening skills and to give them opportunities to advance their home language repertoires.

RhinoSpike (http://www.RhinoSpike.com) is a free site for requesting spoken recordings of texts that are submitted by the user. Teachers can submit a printed text in any language and RhinoSpike will forward that request to a native speaker who will record the text and upload it for access on the RhinoSpike website. Similarly teachers and their students can respond to requests for recordings. English and Spanish are the most widely represented languages at the present time, but many less familiar languages are also listed.

These examples are presented to suggest to readers that it is possible to access full text materials in multiple languages in a short time. Not all languages are available, and not all materials will be suitable for the activity at hand, but teachers are encouraged to invest in the initial explorations of their students' languages to determine what might already be of use to them and their students.

Websites for Language Identification

Many immigrant families speak languages that are not well known and will not be accessible through popular translation and language learning websites. For example, in south Florida, many families come from very rural parts of southern Mexico and Guatemala to work in the agricultural fields. The father may speak enough Spanish to find work and to enroll the children in school, but the language spoken in the home is one of hundreds of Mayan or Oto-Manguen languages. Identifying the language(s) spoken in the home is a critical step for serious efforts to bring home language experiences into the classroom or early childhood setting. The US Office of Head Start has mandated that all children in Head Start programs (Head Start, Early Head Start and Migrant Head Start) be supported in the development of their home languages in addition to English (Improving Head Start for School Readiness Act of 2007). Once the home language has been identified, then language materials can be located and developed for classroom use.

The website Ethnologue (http://www.ethnologue.com) is an encyclopedic reference on the languages of the world. The site features maps of the countries of the world showing the distribution of all known languages and their speakers. Interviewing families with the help of maps, the names of towns and villages and the names of all the language varieties in the region can provide the information necessary to identify a family's language. Once a language has been identified, then language resources can be found through web searches by the language name or the name of the contributing linguist (which is available on Ethnologue). Many linguists whose work has laid the foundation for Ethnologue have published picture dictionaries and other helpful language materials.

For example, a childcare program serving migrant farmworker families in Florida reports that 116 children in their centers speak 'Mixtec' or 'Mixteco' at home (Burns *et al.*, 2012). Mixtec is a language family representing over 52 individual languages, many of which are not mutually intelligible (http://www.ethnologue.com/show_family.asp?subid = 1905-16, http://en.wikipedia.org/wiki/Mixtec_language). Searching for Mixtec language on the internet yields language community webpages (e.g. www.mixteco.org), over 27,000 video clips on YouTube, and no cost print materials such as those posted on linguist Barbara Hallenbach's website (http://www.sil.org/~ hollenbachb/), ranging from a picture dictionary, folktales and songs to grammatical analyses. Many steps remain for the childcare teachers to create meaningful Mixtec language events in their classrooms, but the possibilities are very rich.

Sharing the Workload through Open Educational Resources

The tools and suggested uses presented in this chapter are the beginning steps to creating multilingual assessment and instructional materials for multilingual students. Creating materials that are reliable, accurate and targeted to the instructional objectives of individual students will require significant amounts of time for development and refinement in classroom settings. The same resources that have brought the languages of the world to computers and cell phones have also brought organized networks for open collaboration and product sharing. The Byki language learning website hosts open exchange of shared wordlists (http://www.byki.com/listcentral.html). The Rhinospike website is designed precisely for user requests and open sharing. A global movement to support the identification and dissemination of content-based educational materials was defined in a UNESCO forum in 2002: Open Educational Resources, or OER (http://www.oercommons.org/). Websites devoted to teacher collaboration and shared curricula have followed: Curriki, a K-12 open curricula community (http://www.curriki.org/), MERLOT (Multimedia Educational Resources for Learning and Online Teaching, http://www.merlot.org/merlot/index.htm), and TeachBuzz, a searchable collection of K-12 lesson plans that can be delivered at little or no cost and with no special materials (http://www.teachbuzz.com). These host sites for developing shared curriculum materials offer teachers the opportunity to create multilingual assessment and instructional materials efficiently by collaborating with others – possibilities that apply to a single school or to teachers around the world. At the present time, however, all of these sites are presented in English and all the materials are in English except when designated as 'world language' curricula. I believe that as soon as teachers find their first high quality, content-specific multilingual assessment and instructional materials to use in their classrooms, a multilingual open educational resource movement will expand the availability of these materials very quickly.

Guiding Principles for using Students' Home Languages in Monolingual Instructional Settings

There are classroom settings in which teachers may be restricted in the use of students' home languages in classroom teaching. For example, Arizona, Massachusetts and California all have some form of prohibition against bilingual education at the present time, and many school districts in the United States have adopted a curriculum model that specifies specific blocks of time for intensive English language instruction. The use of home languages in the classroom is discouraged in these settings. One can imagine political conflicts anywhere in the world as a potential source of prohibitions against using certain languages in the classroom. Teachers who find themselves in linguistically restricted teaching environments can still cultivate learning advantages for their multilingual students even if multilingual materials are not acceptable in the classroom. Multilingual materials can be sent home with students. A home visit from the teacher or a community volunteer could guide parents and students on ways to use these materials. Teachers must carefully review the policies of their schools to find opportunities for flexibility in the use of instructional methods and materials. Clark (2009) describes the many instructional models in the US that fall under a general heading of 'structured English immersion' and provides the definition that was presented to voters in Massachusetts: 'Nearly all classroom instruction is in English but with the curriculum and presentation designed for children who are learning the language' (Massachusetts Department of Education, 2003: 7 as cited in Clark, 2009: 43). Language immersion typically means that the learner is immersed in a new language without systematic access to his familiar language. However, the little bit of flexible instructional space that is allowed by the deliberate use of 'nearly entirely' can be a portal for students to be strategically supported with home language materials. If appropriate multilingual assessment and instructional materials are made available to students as part of their regular learning activities, the student may be learning in two languages while the teacher teaches only in one language.

Most linguistically restrictive policies are intended to support students' mastery of the target language – a goal shared by all educators. So the guiding principles for the use of multilingual materials in the classroom are outlined below.

Design multilingual assessment and instructional materials to support students' acquisition of the language of instruction

Materials that bridge students' understanding of how their home language is like and unlike the new language are effective support for second language acquisition. These materials are necessarily multilingual: alphabets, vocabularies, pronunciation activities, grammar comparisons. Furthermore, all education policy makers have the intention of supporting academic success, which leads to the second guiding principle, outlined below.

Design multilingual assessment and instructional materials to support students' mastery of subject area content

A teacher's job is to provide instruction in the objectives of the curriculum, so it is important to focus on creating multilingual materials to support the academic needs of students. Multilingual materials should reflect the subject matter, factual information, demonstrations of knowledge and interpretations of events. Contemporary learning theories recognize that multiple representations of knowledge reflect deeper mastery of learning, and that multiple representations of information are necessary to meet the needs of diverse learners (Jonassen, 1994). By making multilingual assessment and instructional materials available to students in multilingual classrooms, teachers are not teaching in any language other than the language of instruction; however, the teacher is guiding students to make strategic use of all of their cognitive and linguistic resources, including family involvement, in meeting the standard curriculum learning objectives.

Teachers who keep these first two principles in mind will be able to articulate the purpose of multilingual assessment and instructional resources in the classroom to their education team members, administrators, families and other community members. Monolingual members of the school community may better understand what it is like to be growing up with two or more languages when presented with a list of helpful teaching practices for multilingual students. Such a list might include:

- bilingual vocabulary, flashcards for home and school;
- bilingual books for home and school;
- visuals and graphic organizers to reduce the language load, clarify concepts;
- comprehension checks in L1 to ensure understanding;
- L1 rehearsal for L2 speaking and writing presentations;
- resource books and materials in L1 for home and school.

A third principle for using multilingual materials in the classroom is outlined below.

Display multilingual materials in recognition of linguistic diversity in the school community

The connections between language and identity are powerful, and when schools attempt to motivate rapid learning of the instructional language by discouraging the presence of community languages, they inadvertently send an unwelcoming message to multilingual families and students. Social–emotional well-being and parent involvement are critical components of a student's academic success. One way that schools can guard against unintentionally unwelcoming messages is to deliberately create welcoming ones. Based on research in family involvement in schools, Mayer and Cepeda (2007) developed a free, downloadable Spanish-English bilingual book titled *Tomasito's Mother Goes to School/La Mamá de Tomasito Visita la Escuela*. In this story, Tomasito's mother surprises second-grade Tomasito when she interrupts his class to call out to him, using her loud voice and speaking Spanish, that she has brought the library book that he left in the car. Tomasito feels angry and embarrassed, and later, he hurts his mother's feelings. But Tomasito's teacher explains to him that she is very happy to see his mother and that she likes to speak with his mother – in Spanish or English. The story is published by the Harvard Family Research Project with additional support materials on how to use the book to reach out to families, teachers and schools to open multilingual lines of communication (http://www.hfrp/family-involvement/publications-&-resources/tomasito's-mother-comes-to-school/La-mama-visita-la-escuela/).

Schools and the classrooms within them can reflect a deliberately supportive philosophy of bilingualism through institutional signage in different languages as well as student-created multilingual materials. Multilingual greetings, posters, maps, information –visible acknowledgement of students' language backgrounds – are appropriate in every school regardless of the instructional model being implemented.

Always anchor early literacy assessment and instruction to vocabulary, stories, songs and conversational patterns that are well-known to the individual child

Learning to read and write in the language of instruction is an important instructional goal of all early education programs. In these programs, children are systematically exposed to print materials that are matched with pictures, stories, songs and games. Children practice writing, identifying printed words, and increasing their conceptual vocabulary (colors, numbers, shapes, patterns, animals, foods, family, weather, etc.). All models of literacy instruction strategically link familiar language experiences to their printed representations. Young children who are not familiar with the language of the classroom will not be able to attach the same kinds of meaning to print as will their peers who have been speaking the classroom language throughout their early years. Teachers can bring words from students' home languages into early literacy activities to provide opportunities for all students to experience meaningful connections between print and their oral language experience.

As learning to read depends on mapping meaning onto symbolic representations, an important principle of literacy instruction is to ensure that learners know the meanings of what is represented in print. One traditional method for supporting meaning in learning to read is matching pictures to printed words, e.g. picture of a cat accompanied by the written word for 'cat'. This is the basic design principle of picture dictionaries, flash cards, alphabet books, posters and word identification worksheets. A popular teacher education textbook series, *Words Their Way*, offers a Spanish-English illustrated alphabet booklet, a set of illustrations of basic concepts, and word lists in six languages in their volume *Words Their Way with English Language Learners*. The authors of this text (Helman *et al.*, 2012) have provided a strong teaching model that demonstrates the critical importance of linking print to the words that are familiar to students as a bridge to their learning to recognize printed words in English.

Support efforts at every level of instruction to develop and implement multilingual assessment practices for student placement and evaluation of student achievement

As teachers explore the use of multilingual materials for classroom instruction and assessment, they will cultivate the knowledge base that can effectively support improvements to linguistically limited policies and practices in schools. Teachers' language awareness and multilingual instructional efforts will drive improvements in accurate home language identification and education experience at the time of students' enrollment. Accurate identification of a student's home language will support improvements in assessment policies and multilingual procedures for placing students in classrooms based on their target language proficiency, home language proficiency (including reading and writing), and academic knowledge and skills. Appropriate placement of students supports high quality instruction. Teachers do not need to spend weeks and months discovering each student's linguistic and academic profiles if this information is provided when the student enters the class, and instruction can be meaningfully differentiated in ways that include home language materials. As students matriculate through a school's program, multilingual assessment and instructional procedures are likely to be more sensitive and useful in making programmatic decisions such as identifying gifted and talented learners and students with learning or reading difficulties. The recognition that linguistically diverse students are learners in at least two languages, regardless of how monolingual the learning environment may be, makes the need for multilingual assessments obvious. Teachers with experience in creating and using multilingual materials for instruction and informal assessments can provide critical support in programmatic efforts to develop multilingual assessment policies and procedures.

Conclusions

The suggestions for using multilingual assessment and instructional materials in classroom teaching presented in this chapter are not simple, quick fixes to the challenges of teaching in a multilingual setting. Much remains to be done before teachers can conveniently access a test, a vocabulary list, or an illustrated text that is accurately matched to the language of the student and the objectives of the curriculum. Even when these conveniences become more readily available, bilingual support for student learning is not a form of bilingual education that aims to graduate students who are academically proficient in two languages. Students, their families and their communities will determine the home language proficiency of bilingual students in monolingual-instruction schools. What I have presented is a case for the current feasibility of using students' home languages to support informal assessment and instruction, to provide a home language bridge for students to reach new subjects and skills in a new language.

The goal of this chapter has been to raise awareness in classroom teachers of issues associated with the bilingual child's level of proficiency in each of his/her languages and to promote these practitioners' confidence in using assessment and instructional materials in unfamiliar languages for specific, strategic classroom applications. To this end I have described how a teacher might make use of free, online programs and materials to create multilingual assessments for classroom use. An Appendix is provided listing these and other websites that can be of use. Five guiding principles for the use of multilingual assessment and instructional materials in monolingual instructional settings have been presented to provide the rationale that teachers will need to reassure themselves, the larger school community and the community at large that their efforts will ultimately enhance student achievement in the school's language and curriculum.

Key to making multilingual assessment and instructional resources available for every teacher in every school setting is the use of Open Educational Resource platforms in collaborative groups that range from small, school-specific teams to large, global teams with common assessment and instructional needs. Such platforms are quite limited in the K-12, multilingual content that is currently available; however, the potential for these sites to host free K-12 instructional and evaluative materials in the languages of the world is unlimited.

Acknowledgment

The author wishes to thank Deborah Cordier for invaluable discussions of chapter drafts and her extensive knowledge of and commitment to Open Educational Resources.

References

Agirdag, O. (2009) All languages welcome here. *Educational Leadership* 66 (27), 20–25.

Aleman, D., Johnson Jr., J. and Perez, L. (2009) Winning schools for ELLs. *Educational Leadership* 66 (27), 66–69.

Burns, R., Norton, P., Burleson, J. and Chappa, I. (2012, June) Identifying and supporting the indigenous home languages of dual-language learners in Head Start programs. Poster session presented at the meeting of the National Head Start Research Conference, Washington, D.C.

Clark, K. (2009) The case for sheltered English immersion. *Educational Leadership* 66 (27), 42–46.

Coelho, E. (2006) Out of the box: Sharing space with English. *Essential Teacher* 3 (1), 28–31.

Cordier, D. (2011) A partnership for learning: Adult learners in Malawi create a literacy manual. Unpublished proposal submitted for the Fulbright African Regional Research Award.

Danzak, R.L. (2011a) Defining identities through multiliteracies: ELL teens narrate their immigration experiences as graphic stories. *Journal of Adolescent and Adult Literacy* 55, 187–196.

Danzak, R.L. (2011b) The interface of language proficiency and identity: A profile analysis of bilingual adolescents and their writing. *Language, Speech, and Hearing Services in Schools* 42, 506–519.

Danzak, R.L. and Silliman, E.R. (2005) Does my identity speak English? A pragmatic approach to the social world of an English language learner with language impairment. *Seminars in Speech and Language* 26, 189–200.

Genesee, F., Savage, R., Erdos, C. and Haigh, C. (2013) Identification of reading difficulties in students schooled in a second language. In V.C.M. Gathercole (ed.) *Solutions for the Assessment of Bilinguals* (pp. 10–35). Bristol: Multilingual Matters.

Helman, L., Bear, D., Templeton, S., Invernizzi, M. and Johnston, F. (2012) *Words their Way with English Learners: Word Study for Phonics, Vocabulary, and Spelling* (2nd edn). Old Tappan, N.J: Pearson Education.

Hornberger, N.H. and Link, H. (2012) Translanguaging and transnational literacies in multilingual classrooms: A biliteracy lens. *International Journal of Bilingual Education and Bilingualism* 15 (3), 261–278.

Improving Head Start for School Readiness Act of 2007, Pub. L. No. (110-134), (2007)

Jonassen, D.H. (1994) Thinking technology: Toward a constructivist design model. *Educational Technology* 34(4), 34–37.

League of the United Latin American Citizens (LULAC) *et al.* v. State Board of Education Consent Decree, United States District Court for the Southern District of Florida, August 14, 1990. Retrieved from http://www.fldoe.org/aala/cdpage2.asp

Mayer, E. and Cepeda, J. (Illustrator) (2007) Tomasito's mother comes to school/La mamá de Tomasito visita la escuela. Cambridge, MA: Harvard Family Research Project. Retrieved from http://www.hfrp.org/family-involvement/publications-resources/tomasito-s-mother-comes-to-school-la-mama-de-tomasito-visita-la-escuela

Thomas, W.P. and Collier, V.P. (2002) *A National Study of School Effectiveness for Language Minority Students' Long-term Academic Achievement.* Santa Cruz, CA: Center for Research on Education, Diversity and Excellence, University of California, Santa Cruz. Retrieved from http://www.crede.ucsc.edu/research/llaa/1.1_final.html

Appendix: Additional Internet Resources for Multilingual Educational Materials

Online translators, transliterators

FoxLingo, http://www. foxlingo.com. This freeware tool is a meta-translator, linked to many free online translators, and runs only on a Firefox browser (an open source browser that does not collect user data for commercial purposes). Foxlingo supports 75 languages, features links to language learning sites and to language service sites such as text-to-speech.

FreeTranslation, http://freetranslation.com. This free translation program is an extension of a for-profit business specializing in global communication and marketing. It currently translates 30 languages, but is notable for its distinctions between regional varieties of languages: Brazilian and European Portuguese, and Mexican, Latin American and European Spanish. In addition to automatic back-translation switching, the website offers several free tools for translating websites and popular mobile applications.

Google Translate, http://translate.google.com. This free translation program currently supports more than 64 languages. The program features a back-translation switch, a synonym provider, an alternate translation switch, and a highlighting feature that indicates what part of the translation is affected by changes in the input.

imTranslate, http://imtranslator.com. This free translation program currently features text-to-speech functions for English, Chinese, German, Italian, Japanese, Korean, Portuguese, Russian and Spanish in addition to automatic translation for over 50 languages, an automatic back-translation function, and several keyboard/character options.

Language information websites

Ethnologue: Languages of the world, http://ethnologue.com/web.asp. Ethnologue is a free, searchable online dataset of the world's languages and their speakers. The site features detailed language maps and extensive bibliographies of the source materials. The information in the database is the largest known collection of language information, representing the work of thousands of linguists over the last century. One important feature of this resource is the free, downloadable data tables that the public may incorporate into their own database applications using the unique 3-letter language codes developed with the International Organization for Standardization (ISO).

OLAC Language Resource Catalog, http://search.language-archives. org/index.html. The Open Language Archives Community (OLAC) catalog provides free access to information on thousands of languages including texts, audio recordings, dictionaries and grammars, and software.

Omniglot: The online encyclopedia of writing systems and languages, http://omniglot.com. Detailed presentations of the writing systems of more than 180 languages are the main focus of this extensive website. The site also features useful phrases in more than 150 languages with many audio recordings. This all free website is maintained by its developer, Simon Ager, who lives in Bangor, Wales, and blogs about his language learning experiences.

Wikipedia, http://wikipedia.org. This collaboratively edited internet encyclopedia hosts more language information pages than can be enumerated. Each language entry varies in depth and technical detail, but a typical entry provides an outline of the phonology, morphology, and syntax of the language with hyperlinks to related Wikipedia pages for country, region, demographic, culture and other relevant information.

Multimedia websites

OLAC Language Resource Catalog, http://search.language-archives. org/index.html. The Open Language Archives Community (OLAC) catalog, described above, features language audio, video and software resources in an open exchange platform.

RhinoSpike: Foreign Language Audio on Demand, http://www.rhino-spike.com. This free online language learning community tool allows users to request audio recordings by native speakers of specific texts and to share custom-made recordings.

YouTube, http://www.youtube.com. This free video-sharing website has been growing rapidly since its beginning in late 2005. Video submissions come from all over the world, and as such represent the languages of YouTube viewers. The site is searchable by language names.

Language learning websites

Byki, http://byki.com. This website offers free, downloadable interactive flashcards (target language, English gloss, image) in over 70 languages. The flashcard presentation follows a programmed sequence of learning stages, engages listening as well as reading skills, and allows learners to track their progress. The List Central feature of this website allows users to collaborate through the open exchange of lists, expanding the number of available languages and curriculum-appropriate materials.

Foreign Service Institute Language Courses, http://www.fsi-language-courses.org. This site hosts the audio and text materials for the language courses developed by the U.S. Foreign Service Institute that have fallen under public domain. The site currently lists 43 languages. The site is a private, non-profit, volunteer effort with no government affiliation.

Livemocha, http://livemocha.com. This free language learning website offers multi-leveled language instruction in a variety of formats for 38 languages. Learners engage in reading, writing, listening and speaking activities to earn 'tokens' to access more lessons. The site hosts volunteers to interact with learners at no charge.

Spanish Dictionary, Learn Spanish, http://spanishdict.com/learn/. This website offers a free online Spanish language course that features video materials, grammar lessons, speaking exercises, opportunities to link up with others through social media and a point-tracking system for completion of activities. Teachers of native Spanish speakers learning English can 'reverse engineer' the lessons to support English language skills for Spanish speakers.

Support for Elementary Educators through Distance Education in Spanish (SEEDS) http://seeds.coedu.usf.edu/index.htm. This free access website features three modules designed for current practicing generalist elementary school teachers. The first module provides multi-media Spanish language lessons with instructions in English or Spanish. The second module provides teacher resrouces on language acquisition, curriculum and assessment principles for students learning a new language, and other aspects of professional development. The third module presents dual language content area instructional units and lesson plans with resource materials provided. All modules can be downloaded and used as CD-rom material. Most of the activities consist of printable materials, but many pictures, audio and video resources are also provided.

Children's websites

Chillola.com: Where children love language and learn about each other, http://www.chillola.com. This all-free website currently supports basic vocabulary and early learning concepts in English, Spanish, French, German and Italian. Targeted toward young children, the graphics, pictures and activities are bright and appealing. All audio sources are provided by native speakers.

International Children's Digital Library: A library for the world's children, http://en.childrenslibrary.org. In development since 2002, this site features thousands of digitized children's books in many languages and from many countries. The database is searchable by country/region, content type, emotional quality, intended age group and language. Books are presented in their original language with copyright permission from publishers or authors. Users can register to save preferences. The website itself is available in English, Spanish, French, Magyar and Russian.

Mamalisa's World: International Music and Culture, http://mamalisa. com. This site features children's songs, nursery rhymes, poetry, recipes, holidays and games from all over the world. Print materials are presented in English and in their native languages. Some audio and video files are also available.

Piccolingo: Campaign for Early Foreign Language Learning, http://www.piccolingo.pauservers.com. Launched in 2011, the Piccolingo Campaign is a European Commission initiative to help parents understand the benefits of early language learning. The multilingual website provides links to resources and news of Piccolingo Campaign events all around Europe. The Piccolingo YouTube channel currently hosts 234 videos.

Shared curriculum websites

Curriki: K-12 Open Curricula Community, http://www.curriki.org. This free, searchable database of instructional materials features print and multimedia curricula in a variety of formats (lesson plans, units, courses, texts). 'Language' is one of the search features on this site. Quality is maintained by in-house reviewers. This platform supports teacher collaboration through online tools for sharing and editing.

MERLOT (Multimedia Educational Resources for Learning and Online Teaching), http://www.merlot.org/merlot/index.htm. This site focuses on secondary and post secondary education resources including technical trade curricula (e.g. fire safety, health technician). Quality of materials is maintained by reviewers who must undergo a reviewer training course. Communities are organized by discipline or more flexibly by institutional group, and individual user pages are available. Multilingual materials are currently available only through the World Languages resources.

TeachBuzz: Lessons for Anywhere, http://www.teachbuzz.com. This free, searchable database of lesson plans is designed for global applications: lesson plans that can be taught with no special materials or resources. All lessons are currently in English, but because of the open share design, teachers could collaboratively develop lessons in different languages and lessons about different languages. The site maintains the quality of its lesson plans by monitoring the ratings that lesson plans are given by users and by generating lessons written by in-house experts.

Wiki Educator, http://wikieducator.org. This free, collaborative curriculum website features specialized training in using wiki editing tools, customizable user pages, interest clusters and planning initiatives. Print and multimedia materials for preschool through adult and professional development are available. The site is formatted like Wikipedia, with language options in other languages shown in the left column. Only 6 language options are currently available, and little of the content that is available on the English page is available; however, a built-in online translator is available.

8 Assessing Multilingual Students' Writing Skills in Basque, Spanish and English

Jasone Cenoz, Eli Arozena and Durk Gorter

This chapter focuses on the assessment of writing skills in an educational setting in which Basque, Spanish and English are taught, but Basque, a minority language, is the main medium of instruction. The chapter starts by looking at bilingual programs involving regional minority languages and highlights their dual role as both immersion and language maintenance programs. Then it focuses on bi/multilingual education in the Basque Country and its assessment. The results of a study on the acquisition of writing skills in Basque, Spanish and English are reported. Participants were 57 secondary school students with Basque as the main language of instruction and either Basque or Spanish as their first language. The analyses compare the scores obtained in the three languages by students grouped according to their L1s. The results are discussed as related to the characteristics of the multilingual education program and the specific sociolinguistic context of Basque as a minority language.

Introduction

This chapter focuses on the assessment of writing skills in an educational setting in which Basque, Spanish and English are taught, but Basque, a minority language, is the main medium of instruction. Assessment is an integral part of learning and teaching in school contexts in general, and particularly in those in which some students have a second language as the medium of instruction. In this chapter, assessment in Basque schools will be discussed both as related to general evaluations of key subjects such as the PISA assessment, and specific assessment of competencies in the three languages. Moreover, language assessment will include not only separate competences in each of the languages but also combined indexes of bilingualism and multilingualism.

Bilingual education can provide the opportunity to learn new languages, either second languages spoken in the community or foreign languages. Bilingual education can also be an opportunity for some children to develop minority languages spoken as a first language. In the case of minority languages, instruction through the minority language is sometimes limited to the first years of primary school and then there is a shift to a majority language, which becomes the main vehicle of instruction (Gorter & Van der Meer, 2008). The situation with Basque is different: The role of Basque in education has undergone important changes in the last decades. Basque was banned from education for several decades in the 20th century, but political and social changes in the late 1970s and 1980s changed this situation. A strong policy to protect the language and an increase in its status in the last decades has resulted in Basque becoming the main language of instruction in primary and secondary schools all over the Basque Autonomous Community.

In this chapter we first look at immersion programs and language maintenance programs as different types of bilingual education programs, and we examine how these programs are implemented in the Basque Country. Then we look at the specific characteristics of bilingual programs with respect to the use of Basque and Spanish as languages of instruction and at the increasing presence of English in the curriculum. The subsequent section focuses on the assessment of multilinguals and the need to consider different bilingual groups in relation to their first language. We also highlight the importance of looking at all the languages in the speaker's linguistic repertoire when conducting research on bi/multilingualism.

Immersion programs and language maintenance education

Canadian immersion programs constitute a specific type of bilingual education aimed at pupils with English as their L1 and French as their L2. Typically, immersion programs of this type use the L2 as the language of instruction in contexts in which the L1 is strongly supported (Swain & Johnson, 1997: 6–8). There are different types of immersion programs, such as early immersion, late immersion and partial or total immersion, depending on the extent of use of the L2 in the curriculum (Genesee, 1987; Swain & Lapkin, 1982). The aim of these programs is to achieve a higher level of proficiency in the L2 than in traditional programs in which the L2 is taught as a school subject. Immersion programs of this type have spread to many other countries in the world, including European regions where a minority language is spoken, such as Catalonia or the Basque Country (see for example, Cummins & Hornberger, 2008).

Another type of bilingual education program is language maintenance education in the minority language. There are many examples of the success of teaching through indigenous minority languages in different countries. For example, McCarty (2008) discusses the use of languages such as Hawaiian, a Polynesian language, or Navajo, a Native American/Amerindian language, alongside English in bilingual programs in North America. Other examples are the use of Māori as the language of instruction in New Zealand (see for example May & Hill, 2005) or the development of Intercultural Bilingual Education in Latin America, with different native languages used as the medium of instruction (López & Sichra, 2007). The aim of these programs is to develop the minority language and to promote academic success by using the children's first language. These minority languages can then be used for higher level functions both in speaking and in writing.

According to May (2008: 20), bilingual education necessarily 'involves instruction in two languages'. In a strict sense this categorization would not treat educational systems in which only the minority language is used as the language of instruction (as, for example, in Catalan or Basque schools) as bilingual education. However, we believe that in the case of minority languages these programs are also bilingual because they aim at the child's acquiring full proficiency in the majority and the minority language. The majority language is only a school subject but it is very strong outside the school. The fact that the subject 'Spanish language' follows the same curriculum in these regions as in other parts of Spain indicates that the majority language is strong even though it is just a school subject.

Another type of bilingual education involves two-way immersion or dual language immersion programs (see Baker, 2006: chapter 11; Genesee & Lindholm-Leary, 2007). According to De Jong and Howard (2009: 84), these programs, which have been developed mainly in the US, are additive, because they do not replace the L1 with the L2. Students have both the L1 and L2 as the languages of instruction, and although the idea can be to have approximately the same number of students who have each of the two languages as L1 the balance is not always achieved. Participants in these programs in the USA are often native speakers of English and Spanish-speaking immigrants, but other languages are also used.

There is great variation in the types of bilingual education that can be found in European regions where minority languages are spoken (Gorter & Cenoz, 2012). The European Charter for regional or minority languages defines minority languages as those 'that are traditionally used within a given territory of a state by nationals of that state who form a group numerically smaller than the rest of the state's population and [are] different from the official language(s) of that state' (Council of Europe, 1992).

Minority languages are often spoken by a low number of speakers, as is the case for Basque or Frisian, but there are some exceptions, such as Catalan, which has several million speakers. The language policy to protect and promote the use of minority languages in education varies from region to region, and the use of the minority language in education depends on the strength of those policies. In the case of Catalan and Basque, the policies are strong, so they are used as the language of instruction at all levels of education. For example in Catalonia, Catalan is the language of instruction in over 90% of primary schools (Vila, 2008). A similar trend can be found in Basque education.

Bilingual programs in regions such as Catalonia, Valencia, the Basque Country, Wales or Friesland are at one and the same time immersion programs and language maintenance programs. They are immersion programs in the minority language for children who speak the majority language as a first language (Vila, 2008). School children from Spanish-speaking households are increasingly being taught in the minority language in other regions as well (see Cenoz, 2008; Vila, 2008). This situation is similar to that of children from English-speaking households in Wales when they have Welsh as the medium of instruction (Lewis, 2008) and in Ireland when they attend 'all-Irish schools' (Harris, 2008). Some of these programs are called 'super immersion' because the minority language is used as the language of instruction for all school subjects. Other programs have both the majority and minority languages as languages of instruction, and there are programs with three languages of instruction as well (see Cenoz, 2009; Gorter & van der Meer, 2008).

These bilingual programs are at the same time language maintenance programs for school children who have the minority language as their L1. These children are exposed to the majority language both at school, where they study the majority language as a subject (and in some programs as an additional language of instruction), and in the social context because the majority language is used extensively outside school.

Multilingual education in Basque schools

Schools in the Basque Autonomous community generally have three or four languages in the curriculum. Basque and Spanish are official languages and can be used as languages of instruction as well as being school subjects. A foreign language, generally English, is also compulsory for all students. French, German and Latin can be optional subjects in secondary school.

Basque was recognized as an official language (alongside Spanish) in the Basque Autonomous Community in 1982. At that time, three models of language schooling were established (models A, B and D).

- *A model programs* have Spanish as the language of instruction and Basque as a school subject. Basque is studied as a second language.

- *B model programs* have both Basque and Spanish as languages of instruction, each for approximately 50% of school time, although there is considerable variation from school to school. Basque is also studied as a second language in this model.
- *D model programs* have Basque as the language of instruction and Spanish as a school subject. Although Spanish is only a subject and in many cases the students' second language, the syllabus for Spanish is the same as in the other programs. Spanish is not studied as a second language.

As opposed to the A and B models, which are intended for students with Spanish as their L1, the D model was originally created as a language maintenance program for speakers with Basque as their L1, in order to give such students the opportunity to be taught through their first language. However, a large number of students with Spanish as their first language are in the D model nowadays, so this model is both a language-maintenance program for Basque L1 speakers and an immersion programme for L1 Spanish speakers. This dual function is also shared by dual immersion programs, but there are some important differences. Dual immersion programs are characterized by the use of two languages of instruction and often have students with both languages as L1 (De Jong & Howard, 2009). The D model shares with dual immersion programs the fact that there can be students of the majority and the minority languages in the same class but the D model only has Basque as the language of instruction. The B model could be more similar to dual immersion programs because there are two languages of instruction (Basque and Spanish) but there are differences as well because almost all students in the B model have the majority language as their L1 and this is not the case in dual immersion programs.

The patterns of enrolment in the three types of schools in the Basque country are as shown in Table 8.1. As can be seen in the table, the D model has become the most popular type of school in the Basque Autonomous Community.

The data indicate that most students have Basque as the language of instruction or one of the languages of instruction and this trend has increased

Table 8.1 Registration in pre-primary, primary and secondary school in the Basque Autonomous Community. Academic year 2010–2011 (Basque Government, 2011)

	Language of instruction	Number of students	Percentage
A model	Spanish	58,680	18.9%
B model	Basque and Spanish	69,238	22.3%
D model	Basque	182,465	58.8%
Total		310,383	100

over the years. Parents choose Basque-medium instruction for different reasons (Cenoz, 2009). Basque-speaking parents want their children to develop their first language by having it as the language of instruction and because there is enough exposure to Spanish outside school. Some Spanish-speaking parents of Basque origin have the idea of recovering a language that was in the family spoken by grandparents or great-grandparents but was lost in their own generation because there was no opportunity to use it at school or in other public domains. Other parents feel that as they live in the Basque Country, learning through Basque provides more opportunities, including access to jobs with Basque as a requirement. The distribution among the three models varies according to the location of the school, and the A model (Spanish-medium instruction), with only 18.9% of the students, is not easily found in areas with a higher percentage of Basque speakers.

Most students in the A and B models have Spanish as their first language. However, in the last years the number of speakers of other languages has increased owing to immigration and now almost 7% of the students in schools in the Basque Autonomous Community are immigrants (see also Etxeberria & Elosegi, 2008). About half of these immigrants can speak Spanish because they come from Latin America (mainly from Colombia, Bolivia and Ecuador), but others come from African and European countries (Morocco, Romania, Bulgaria). Immigrant students are enrolled in the three models, but they tend to enroll more in models A and B than in the D model (Etxeberria & Elosegi, 2008).

Apart from the values associated with the acquisition and maintenance of both Basque and Spanish in the Basque Country, the ability to speak English is also perceived as an important tool in Basque society. In most schools, as a result, English is taught from the age of four, and some schools also teach one or two subjects through the medium of English.

The fact that a minority language, Basque, has become the main language of instruction all over the Basque Autonomous Community has led to research studies and evaluations on language and academic development (Cenoz, 2009). In the next section some aspects of assessment will be discussed.

The assessment of multilingual education

Assessment is an essential part of the teaching process, and one of the challenges of research in bilingual education in the last decades has been to document that bilinguals are not at a disadvantage in their overall achievement at school (Baker, 2006). The idea that bilingualism could be a burden for cognitive development is no longer accepted, but it is nevertheless still important to demonstrate the efficacy of bilingual programs. This is even more pressing in the case of minority languages that do not have a strong tradition as languages of instruction. Teaching through these languages poses challenges regarding the development of materials and the use of a minority language for academic purposes (see Zalbide & Cenoz, 2008). As Rau (2005: 410) notes in relation to Māori-medium programs, assessment is crucial for confirming achievement to different stakeholders, such as educational authorities, educators, the students, and their families.

In the Basque Country assessment is a major concern for a number of reasons. First, external evaluations of school achievement are increasingly common, and reveal the levels of achievements, not only for educational forums but also for the society at large. Among these evaluations, the most well known is PISA (Programme for International Student Assessment). This assessment has been carried out by the OECD (The Organisation for Economic Co-operation and Development) since 2000 and takes place every three years, with students from 65 countries participating in the 2009 evaluation (www.pisa.oecd.org). Another important international evaluation is TIMSS (Trends in International Mathematics and Science Study), undertaken by the International Association for Evaluation of Educational Achievement (IEA), which takes place every four years (almost 60 countries participated in 2007) (http://isc.bc.edu).

Apart from these international evaluations, the Basque Government Department of Education carries out its own diagnostic assessment program, introduced in 2009. Tests are administered every year in the 4th year of primary education (9- to 10-year-old children) and in the second year of secondary education (13- to 14-year-old children). There is also an external exam at the end of secondary education, which is an entrance exam for university studies.

Students in bilingual programs are expected to show at least the same level of achievement as children in non-bilingual programs but their conditions particularly in the case of minority languages are not the same. As Rau (2010) explains, in the case of minority languages there are many teachers who have learned the minority language as a second language and use it as the language of instruction. An additional challenge that teaching through the medium of a minority language faces, which can also have an effect on assessment, is the availability of materials. There are fewer textbooks and even though some electronic resources exist for many minority languages they are not available to the same extent as for majority languages. Other challenges are related to the corpus of the language, which has had to be developed in the last years, particularly in relation to specialized lexicon, and the standardization of the language. The processes of standardization that strong European languages such as English, French or Spanish went through in the XVIIth and XVIIIth centuries with the publication of grammars and dictionaries started in the XXth century in the case of Basque. This is an important issue for language and content assessment in minority languages in school contexts because the gap between academic language and home language may be bigger than in the case of majority languages.

In general terms evaluations of language proficiency carried out in Basque schools indicate that students with more exposure to Basque in Basque-medium instruction models obtain significantly higher scores in Basque, particularly in the D model. There are some differences across the A, B and D models in performance on Spanish, but the students taught through Basque achieve in general a very good command of Spanish, and in many cases Spanish remains their dominant language (see Cenoz, 2009, for a review).

The results related to other areas of the curriculum indicate that students with Basque as the language of instruction can achieve scores similar to (or higher than) those of students with Spanish as the language of instruction. The results of a substantial number of evaluations clearly indicate that socio-economic status is a better predictor of achievement in mathematics or science than having either Basque or Spanish as the language of instruction (ISEI-IVEI 2010b).

The OECD PISA (Programme for International Student Assessment) aims to evaluate educational systems in different parts of the world by testing 15-year-old students. The PISA evaluations started in 2000 and so far over 65 countries and regions have taken part. Table 8.2 shows the results of the most recent PISA assessment for science, mathematics and reading literacy, and compares the average scores in the Basque Autonomous Community, Spain and the OECD (all the countries participating in the evaluation).

For the three measures, the scores in the BAC were higher than the Spanish averages, and the differences were statistically significant for mathematics and reading literacy. Similar results were observed in the 2003 and 2006 PISA evaluations, which indicate that students in Basque bilingual programs perform better than many students who are not in bilingual education in other areas of Spain. As Cenoz (2009: 108) points out when discussing the 2006 results, 'this does not imply a cause–effect relationship but it shows that bilingual education is compatible with successful academic development'.

These results are in agreement with research studies on minority children being educated in the majority language in the US (see for example Genesee & Riches, 2006; McCarty, 2008), in Latin America (López & Sichra, 2008), and in several programs in Asia and Africa (Heugh & Skutnabb Kangas, 2010). They are also compatible with research showing that students in immersion programs learn another language and acquire literacy skills at

Table 8.2 Pisa 2009. Results for the BAC, Spain and OECD

	BAC	Spain	OECD average
Science	495	488	501
Mathematics	510	483	496
Reading literacy	494	481	493

Source: ISEI-IVEI, 2010a

no cost to their overall academic achievement or their first language skills (Genesee, 1987, 2004; Johnson & Swain, 1997; Swain & Lapkin, 1982).

Taking into account the double function of the D model as an immersion program for Spanish L1 speakers and a language maintenance program for Basque L1 speakers, it is also crucial to go beyond the comparison of the models and to focus on the effect of instruction in an L2 on the students' first language. Most research studies and evaluations to date have taken the D model as a whole without differentiating the two groups of students (L1 Basque, L1 Spanish) and have used the 'ideal' native speaker of each of the two languages (Basque and Spanish) as a reference. Evaluations carried out so far indicate that D model students acquire a more balanced type of bilingualism than students in the other models (Cenoz, 2009). However, competence in each of the two languages is also necessarily linked to factors outside the school curriculum. In the D model, Basque L1 students who speak Basque at home, use Basque as the language of instruction, and live in Basque-speaking areas acquire a high level of proficiency in Spanish. However, they may not reach exactly the same level of proficiency in Spanish as other students who use Spanish for all purposes and at all times except for a very limited number of hours of Basque and English lessons at school (see for example Santiago *et al.*, 2008). Conversely, Spanish L1 students in the D model who speak Spanish at home and in everyday communication may not achieve the same level of proficiency in Basque as Basque L1 speakers even if they have Basque as the main language of instruction. Thus, students in the D model may be relatively balanced bilinguals, but their languages are not necessarily 'perfectly' balanced. According to Cook (1995), second language users possess unique forms of competence and should not be seen as the sum of monolinguals. If we adopt this holistic view of multilingual proficiency already proposed by Grosjean (1985) D model students could be evaluated as multilingual speakers who have a linguistic repertoire that is different from that of monolinguals, and they are not expected to be double monolinguals (see also Cenoz & Gorter, 2011).

An important step when considering a holistic view of multilingual proficiency can be to take the students' linguistic repertoire into account including the differences in their L1s. In contexts where a minority language is spoken the L1 children enter the school which is often linked to the sociolinguistic context. For example in Ireland, about half of the schools with Irish as the medium of instruction are located in the Gaeltacht, the traditional Irish-speaking area, and the other half are 'all-Irish' schools located in the rest of the country (Murtagh, 2007). The former are predominantly language-maintenance programs, serving children with Irish as their L1, and the latter are immersion programs. In the case of Wales, the North West, where Welsh is strongest, has more language-maintenance programs than the North East and the South East (see Lewis, 2008). In the Basque Country, Basque is stronger in Bizkaia and Gipuzkoa, and more in smaller towns than cities. Even so, in the Basque context, it is very unusual to have a homogeneous class who share the same L1, and most classes in the D model include immersion and language maintenance students. Furthermore, the linguistic composition of the classes is dynamic and can change over time (Harris, 2008; Lewis 2008).

Some data for Basque language proficiency measured according to children's L1 are now available through the diagnostic assessment program introduced in 2009 by the ISEI-IVEI (2009a, 2009b, 2010b, 2010c). These evaluations were administered to the total population in the grades, which included almost 20,000 students, for the 4th year of primary and for the 2nd year of secondary combined. The Basque language tests were pen and paper tests, one for each level, and measured listening comprehension and written production. Table 8.3 presents the results according to three levels of performance: lower than average, intermediate and advanced.

The data indicate that in both years a higher proportion of Basque L1 students obtained high scores in Basque. This can be expected because Basque L1 students are more likely to use Basque more often and are more exposed to Basque in the family, with friends or through the media. Spanish L1 students who live in a Spanish-speaking environment and have Basque as the language of instruction in the D model have fewer opportunities to use the language. Even though Spanish L1 students have extensive exposure to Basque at school they do not reach the level of students with Basque as their L1 and these results confirm research conducted in Canadian immersion programs (Genesee, 1987).

These differences are particularly important when Basque is the language of instruction because a lower proficiency in Basque could affect overall achievement. Some differences in achievement in mathematics and social science between Basque L1 and Spanish L1 students in the D model are reported in the diagnostic assessment (ISEI-IVEI 2010b, 2010c). These results indicate that Spanish L1 speakers (or speakers of other languages in the case of primary) obtain lower scores than Basque L1 speakers both in

Table 8.3 Proportion of children showing three levels of Basque language proficiency, according to first language and school level

	Lower	*Intermediate*	*Advanced*
4th Primary			
Basque L1	12.1	39.9	48.0
Spanish/other L1	21.4	49.1	29.5
2nd Secondary			
Basque L1	14.6	45.1	40.7
Spanish L1	26.3	47.5	26.2

Source: ISEI-IVEI 2010b, 2010c

mathematics and social science (in both the 4th year of primary and the 2nd year of secondary). Further research is needed to determine if there is a cause–effect relationship between proficiency in Basque and achievement in other subjects because there could be also other variables involved, such as socioeconomic status and socio-educational background.

Another study that distinguishes between Basque L1 and Spanish L1 students was conducted by Sagasta (2003), who focused on the acquisition of writing skills in English as a third language. She reported some significant differences in some writing skills, indicating that Basque L1 students had some advantages over Spanish L1 students when learning English as a third language. She interpreted these results as being linked to the advantages of a more balanced type of Basque-Spanish bilingualism on the part of the Basque L1 learners. In this case the results could be explained as related to proficiency both in Basque and Spanish and not in Basque only. More research is certainly needed to understand the lower performance of Spanish L1 speakers in the D model on both English as an L3 and other content subjects.

An important contribution to the study of proficiency in minority languages has been made by Gathercole et al. (2008) who have developed a receptive vocabulary test for Welsh. It is a norm-referenced test that unlike many other tests, distributes children according to their exposure to Welsh into three groups: 'only Welsh at home', 'Welsh and English at home' and 'only English at home'. The test provides information on 'where the child stands in relation to all children learning the given language, and where the child stands in relation to children with a similar exposure to the language' (Gathercole et al., 2008: 680). This distinction has important implications for Welsh L2 students because they are not compared against the yardstick of Welsh L1 speakers. Welsh L2 speakers' scores are evaluated as compared to the general average, as it is the case in the diagnostic assessment of Basque in Table 8.3, but also as compared to other Welsh L2 speakers.

Another strategy for assessing the viability of programs that have a double function, immersion and language maintenance, such as the D model in the Basque Country, is to assess proficiency in all the languages in the learners' repertoire. This is also done in dual immersion programs (Genesee & Lindholm-Leary, 2008) but in the case of the Basque Country we have the possibility of assessing proficiency in three languages. By assessing proficiency in the different languages and controlling for the influence of the L1 at the same time, it can be possible to obtain a more detailed picture of proficiency.

Writing in Basque, Spanish and English

In this section, we analyze the written production of students in a Basque medium program (D model). The aims of this study were to examine possible differences between Basque L1 and Spanish L1 students in total linguistic repertoire. First we look at general writing skills in each of the three languages. Then, taking a holistic perspective of multilingualism we consider the bilingual and multilingual skills and finally we look at the specific dimensions of writing skills. The research questions were the following:

(1) Are there differences between Basque L1 students and Spanish L1 students when writing in Basque, Spanish and English?
(2) Are there differences in the global level of multilingualism obtained by Basque L1 and Spanish L1 students?
(3) Which are the differences in the specific dimensions of writing in the three languages?

Method

Participants

Participants were 57 secondary school students, 49% of which were male and 51% female. They were in the 3rd year of secondary education (14 to 15 years of age), with a mean age of 14.56. All participants were enrolled in model D schools, with Basque as the language of instruction, and studied Spanish and English as school subjects. For 30% of the participants Basque was their first language; for 70% of the participants Spanish was their first language. The 57 students were from three different schools in the provinces of Gipuzkoa and Araba in the Basque Country.

Materials

Three pictures were used, one for each language. The three pictures included people and animals and they showed different actions. The type of picture was the same for the three languages but the actions were different. One of the pictures showed a picnic area next to a lake where people were relaxing. The second picture was on a farm and the third one in a building where people were engaged in different activities. All the students had the same picture for each of the languages.

Procedure

All participants completed a general background questionnaire and wrote three compositions, one in each language. The compositions were written on different days for each of the languages. Participants were asked to look at the given picture and to describe or tell a story about the people and actions they could observe.

The essays were then evaluated by two different blind evaluators using the ESL Composition Profile developed by Jacobs *et al.* (1981), a widely used scoring rubric that combines holistic and analytic scoring. The essays were scored for five dimensions: content (max = 30), organization (max = 20), vocabulary (max = 20), language use (max = 25), and mechanics (max = 5), with a possible total of 100. The scores are based on a number of descriptors for each of the dimensions. For example the score on language use is based on the following descriptors: effective complex constructions, agreement, tense, number, word order/function, articles, pronouns and prepositions. The score on the mechanics of writing is based on spelling, punctuation, capitalization, paragraphing and handwriting. There are no specific scores for each of the descriptors, only for the five dimensions.

Results

In this section first we give the means and standard deviations for the total scores in each of the languages. Then we proceed to answer the three research questions.

The total scores range from a minimum of 34 points to a maximum of 100. The mean scores for each language overall are shown in Table 8.4.

The means of the writing skills in the three languages indicate that participants achieve a more similar level of proficiency in Basque and Spanish than in English. It is also interesting to observe that the standard deviation for English is higher than for Basque and Spanish, indicating that the scores are less homogeneous.

In order to answer the first research question we compared the total scores obtained by two groups of students (Basque L1 students and Spanish L1 students) in the three languages: Basque, Spanish and English. A t-test analysis was carried out so as to see the differences between the means. The results can be seen in Figure 8.1.

The results of the t-tests indicate that there are significant differences in the general writing scores for two of the languages: Basque (t (55) = 2.11, $p = 0.03$) and English (t (55) = 2.17, $p = 0.03$). The difference for Spanish did not reach significance (t (55) = $- 0.18$, $p = 0.85$). The scores obtained by students with Basque as their L1 are significantly higher than the scores obtained by students with Spanish as their L1 for both Basque and English.

The second research question also aims at analyzing differences between Basque L1 students and Spanish L1 students but not in the three separate languages but in the global measures of bilingualism and multilingualism. This is a different approach because the whole linguistic repertoire is measured at the same time instead of individual languages (see Cenoz & Gorter,

Table 8.4 General scores in writing in Basque, Spanish and English

Max = 100	Mean	S. D.
Basque	87.53	6.49
Spanish	86.09	6.14
English	68.19	11.88

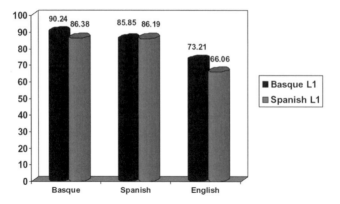

Figure 8.1 Total scores in Basque, Spanish and English (max = 100)

2011). In order to answer this question two indexes were created, one for bilingualism and another one for multilingualism. The bilingualism index is the result of adding up the global scores of Basque and Spanish and the multilingualism index results from adding up the scores of Basque, Spanish and English. The results obtained by Basque L1 students and Spanish L1 students in these indexes can be seen in Figure 8.2.

The results of the *t*-tests indicate that there are no significant differences in the global measure of bilingualism (t (55) = 1.11, $p = 0.27$), and for the differences in the global measure of multilingualism the differences are only marginally significant (t (55) = 1.90, $p = 0.06$).

In order to answer the third research question we looked at the different dimensions of writing proficiency analyzed so as to see the differences between Basque L1 students and Spanish L1 students in more detail. Table 8.5 shows the mean scores in Basque. The third research question aims at analyzing the differences in writing skills in more detail by looking at the different dimensions. A MANOVA analysis was performed in order to test the effect of the two groups (Basque L1 vs. Spanish L1) on the five dimensions of writing (content, organization, vocabulary, language use and mechanics) for the three languages. The results are shown in Table 8.5.

There was a statistically significant difference between students with Basque and Spanish as a first language ($F(1,41) = 2.26, p = 0.01$). Regarding Basque language scores, the results of the Manova indicate that there are significant differences in three of the five dimensions of writing proficiency: vocabulary ($F(1,41) = 5.02$, $p = 0.03$), use of the language ($F(1,41) = 5.82, p = 0.02$) and mechanics ($F(1,41) = 6.51, p = 0.01$). The scores obtained by students with Basque as their L1 are significantly higher than the scores obtained by students with Spanish as their L1 in these three dimensions. There were no significant differences between Basque L1 students and Spanish L1 students in the five dimensions of writing proficiency

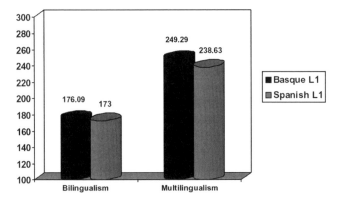

Figure 8.2 Bilingual and multilingual scores

in Spanish. In the case of English, the results of the ANOVA indicate that there are significant differences in three of the five dimensions of writing proficiency: vocabulary $(F(1,41) = 12.63, p = 0.00)$, use of the language $(F(1,41) = 5.02, p = 0.03)$ and mechanics $(F(1,41) = 6.19, p = 0.01)$. The scores

Table 8.5 Results in the specific dimensions of writing in Basque, Spanish and English

	Basque L1	Spanish L1	F-value	Significance
	Mean SD	Mean SD		
Basque				
Content	26.88 2.12	26.80 2.22	002	0.89
Organization	18.71 1.05	17.95 1.66	2.99	0.09
Vocabulary	17.82 0.63	16.80 1.83	5.02	0.03*
Use	22.00 1.62	20.42 2.47	5.82	0.02*
Mechanics	4.82 0.39	4.40 0.63	6.51	0.01*
Spanish				
Content	26.35 2.34	26.83 1.78	0.69	0.41
Organization	17.82 1.74	17.80 1.30	0.00	0.95
Vocabulary	16.94 1.75	17.20 1.34	0.37	0.55
Use	20.47 2.29	20.67 1.71	0.14	0.71
Mechanics	4.35 0.78	4.03 0.66	2.63	0.11
English				
Content	23.12 3.69	21.88 3.76	1.31	0.26
Organization	15.82 2.58	15.28 3.08	0.41	0.52
Vocabulary	14.41 2.37	12.18 2.08	12.63	0.00*
Use	17.00 3.77	14.50 3.77	5.02	0.03*
Mechanics	4.00 0.93	3.37 0.84	6.19	0.01*

obtained by students with Basque as their first languages are significantly higher than the scores obtained by students with Spanish as their L1 in these three dimensions.

Discussion

In this chapter we have looked at language proficiency in writing in three languages, Basque, Spanish and English. The data come from a specific bilingual program in which Basque, a minority language, is used as the language of instruction. But they can have implications for assessment of other languages and other bilingual and multilingual programs as well.

The results regarding the first research question, whether there are differences between Basque L1 students and Spanish L1 students when writing in Basque, Spanish and English, indicate that Basque L1 students obtained significantly better scores in Basque and English, but that there were no significant differences between groups in Spanish. The better results in Basque by Basque L1 speakers can be expected, because these speakers usually have more opportunities to use Basque outside school and tend to live in areas where more Basque is spoken. Even though Basque is the language of instruction for all subjects (except English and Spanish) Spanish L1 students do not reach the same level of Basque as their Basque L1 classmates. For many of these Spanish L1 students Basque is the school language but not their main language of communication and they even use Spanish at school when talking to other classmates.

The fact that no significant differences were found in Spanish can be explained as related to the situation of Basque as a minority language. Even Basque L1 speakers with Basque as the language of instruction who study Spanish only as a subject can acquire a high level of proficiency in Spanish. These students are exposed to Spanish in a context in which everybody is fluent in Spanish and only some people (around 30% for the whole of the Basque Country) are fluent in Basque.

The results for English confirm those obtained by Sagasta (2003), but they are more difficult to explain. Sagasta (2003) reported the higher results of Basque L1 speakers in terms of the level of bilingualism in Basque and Spanish participants had. Basque L1 speakers were considered to be more balanced bilinguals than Spanish L1 speakers.

However, our results obtained regarding our second research question do not confirm that Basque L1 students are more balanced bilinguals than Spanish L1 students. There are no significant differences between the two groups in the global level of bilingualism and only marginally significant differences in the global level of multilingualism. Therefore, these results indicate that when considering only Basque writing skills there are differences between Basque L1 and Spanish L1 speakers, but if we look at the whole linguistic repertoire as suggested by holistic approaches (Cook, 1995; Grosjean, 1985) there are no differences. The measurement of bilingual and multilingual skills offers a different perspective because it compares different types of multilingual students rather than native vs. non-native students for each of the languages. The data presented here are limited to a specific context and more research is necessary to analyze the characteristics of different types of multilinguals controlling for more factors and using larger samples.

The results relative to the third research question, concerning the differences in the specific dimensions of writing in the three languages, indicate, as can be expected from the general scores, that there are some significant differences in Basque and English but not in Spanish. It is interesting to see that the significant differences are in vocabulary, language use and the mechanics of writing and not in content and organization. A possible explanation is that content and organization are cognitive and academic and can be transferred more easily across languages. When a student makes some progress when learning to write a relevant text and is learning how to write his/her ideas clearly or how to link them appropriately in one language, there is the possibility of using these resources in another language. This cognitive academic transfer was reported by Idiazabal and Larringan (1997), who conducted a study in the Basque Country with D model students. In that study an experimental group had a specific intervention to improve the writing of argumentative texts in Basque while the control group went on with their ordinary Basque language classes. At the end of the study, the argumentative texts produced by the experimental group scored better than those of the control group not only in Basque, as was expected, but also in Spanish. Students had transferred the skills they had acquired from Basque to Spanish. The results of the study reported in this chapter do not show any significant differences between Basque L1 and Spanish L1 students in content and organization for any of the languages, and it could be argued that these cognitive academic dimensions are shared in the three languages. On the other hand, the significant differences in the more linguistic dimensions (vocabulary, use of the language, mechanics) can be related to the specific aspects of the languages that cannot be shared so easily.

In this chapter we have highlighted the importance of considering the whole linguistic repertoire of students in bilingual programs. They should be considered as multilingual speakers, not persons who will necessarily achieve the competence of an 'ideal' native speaker of each of the languages. The results of this study also show that we can have a different picture when assessment looks at each language at a time or at global bilingual or multilingual proficiency. Language assessment in bilingual and multilingual programs could certainly benefit from a 'Focus on Multilingualism', understood as 'an approach that looks at the whole linguistic repertoire of multilingual speakers and language learners and at the relationships between the languages when conducting research, teaching or assessing different languages' (Cenoz & Gorter, 2011). Another important finding to take into account is the sociolinguistic context, particularly in the case of minority languages, so as to explain, along with educational variables, the similarities and differences in students' proficiency. In this chapter, language assessment has been related to the learner's linguistic repertoire; the results indicate that multilingual competence is complex and different from competence in each of the languages. Assessment in school contexts should take this complexity into account and should consider its implications for the future of multilingual learners.

Acknowledgments

This research was carried out with the assistance of the Spanish Ministry of Economy and Competiveness research grants EDU2009-11601/ EDU2012-32191 and the Basque Department of Education, Research and Universities IT-714-13 (UFI 11/54).

References

Baker, C. (2006) *Foundations of Bilingual Education and Bilingualism* (4th edn). Clevedon: Multilingual Matters.
Basque Government (2011) Department of Education. Retrieved from http:// www.hezkuntza.ejgv.euskadi.net/r43-540/es/
Cenoz, J. (2008) Achievements and challenges in bilingual and multilingual education in the Basque Country. *Aila Review* 21, 13–30.
Cenoz, J. (2009) *Towards Multilingual Education: Basque Educational Research from an International Perspective*. Bristol: Multilingual Matters.
Cenoz, J. and Gorter, D. (2011) Focus on multilingualism: A study of trilingual writing. *The Modern Language Journal* 95 (3), 356–369.
Cook, V. (1995) Multi-competence and the learning of many languages. *Language, Culture and Curriculum* 8, 93–98.
Council of Europe (1992) European Charter for Regional or Minority languages. Retrieved from www.coe.int/t/e/legal_affairs/local_and_regional_democracy/regional_or_ minority_languages/1_The_Charter/_summary.asp
Cummins, J. and Hornberger, N. (eds) (2008) *Encyclopedia of Language and Education. Vol 5. Bilingual Education*. New York: Springer.
De Jong, E.J. and Howard, E.R. (2009) Integration in two-way immersion education: Equalizing linguistic benefits. *International Journal of Bilingual Education and Bilingualism* 12 (1), 81–99.
Etxeberria, F. and Elosegi, K. (2008) Basque, Spanish and immigrant minority languages in the Basque School. *Language, Culture and Curriculum* 21, 69–84.
Gathercole, V.C.M., Thomas, E.M. and Hughes, E. (2008) Designing a normed receptive vocabulary test for bilingual populations: A model from Welsh. *International Journal of Bilingual Education and Bilingualism* 11, 678–720.
Genesee, F. (1987) *Learning Through Two Languages: Studies of Immersion and Bilingual Education*. Cambridge, MA: Newbury House.
Genesee, F. (2004) What do we know about bilingual education for majority-language students. In T.K. Bhatia and W.C. Ritchie (eds) *The Handbook of Bilingualism* (pp. 547–576). London: Blackwell.

Genesee, F. and Lindholm-Leary, K. (2008) Dual language education in Canada and the United States. In J. Cummins and N. Hornberger (eds) *Encyclopedia of Language and Education* (pp. 253–266). New York: Springer.

Genesee, F. and Riches, C. (2006) Literacy. Instructional issues. In F. Genesee, K. Lindholm-Leary, W.M. Saunders and D. Christian (eds) *Educating English Language Learners: A Synthesis of Research Evidence* (pp. 109–175). New York: Cambridge University Press.

Gorter, D. and Cenoz, J. (2012) Regional minorities, education and language revitalization. In M. Martin-Jones, A. Blackledge and A. Creese (eds) *Routledge Handbook of Multilingualism* (pp. 184–198). London: Routledge.

Gorter, D. and Van der Meer, C. (2008) Developments in bilingual Frisian-Dutch education in Friesland. *Aila Review* 21, 87–103.

Grosjean, F. (1985) The bilingual as a competent but specific speaker-hearer. *Journal of Multilingual and Multicultural Development* 6, 467–77.

Harris, J. (2008) The declining role of primary schools in the revitalisation of Irish. *Aila Review* 21, 49–68.

Heugh, K. and Skutnabb-Kangas, T. (eds) (2010) *Multilingual Education Works: from the Periphery to the Centre*. Delhi: Orient Blackswan.

Idiazabal, I. and Larringan, L.M. (1997) Transfert de maîtrises discursives dans un programme d'enseignement bilingue basque-espagnol. *AILE. Acquisition et Interaction en Langue Étrangère* 10, 107–126.

ISEI-IVEI (2009a) Ebaluazio Diagnostica-Evaluación Diagnóstica 2009. 2° Curso de Educación Secundaria Obligatoria. Retrieved from www.isei-ivei.net/cast/pub/ED10-ejecutivo/ESO-EJECUTIVO10-Final.pdf

ISEI-IVEI (2009b) Ebaluazio Diagnostica-Evaluación Diagnóstica 2009. 2° Curso de Educación Secundaria Obligatoria. Retrieved from www.isei-ivei.net/cast/pub/ED10-ejecutivo/EJECUTIVO_EP.pdf

ISEI-IVEI (2010a) PISA 2009 Euskadiko Emaitzen Aurkezpena. Presentación de resultados del País Vasco. Retrieved from www.isei-ivei.net/cast/pub/pisa2009/PISA2009_RESULTADOS.pdf

ISEI-IVEI (2010b) Ebaluazio Diagnostica-Evaluación Diagnóstica 2010. 4° Curso de Educación Primaria. Retrieved from www.isei-ivei.net/cast/pub/ED10-ejecutivo/EJECUTIVO_EP.pdf

ISEI-IVEI (2010c) Ebaluazio Diagnostica-Evaluación Diagnóstica 2010. 2° Curso de Educación Secundaria Obligatoria. Retrieved from www.isei-ivei.net/cast/pub/ED10-ejecutivo/ESO-EJECUTIVO10-Final.pdf

Jacobs, H.L., Zingraf, S.A., Wormuth, D.R., Hartfiel, V.F. and Hughey, J.B. (1981) *Testing ESL Composition*. Rowley, MA: Newbury House.

Lewis, G. (2008) Current challenges in bilingual education in Wales. *Aila Review* 21, 69–86.

López, L.E. and Sichra, I. (2008) Intercultural bilingual education among indigenous peoples in Latin America. In J. Cummins and N. Hornberger (eds) *Encyclopedia of Language and Education. Vol 5. Bilingual Education* (pp. 295–309). New York: Springer.

May, S. (2008) Bilingual/Immersion education: what the research tells us. In J. Cummins and N. Hornberger (eds) *Encyclopedia of Language and Education. Vol 5. Bilingual Education* (pp. 19–34). New York: Springer.

May, S. and Hill, R. (2005) Maori-medium education: Current issues and challenges. *International Journal of Bilingual Education and Bilingualism* 8, 377–403.

McCarty, T.L. (2008) Bilingual education by and for American Indians, Alaska natives and native Hawaiians. In J. Cummins and N. Hornberger (eds) *Encyclopedia of Language and Education. Vol 5. Bilingual Education* (pp. 239–251). New York: Springer.

Murtagh, L. (2007) Out-of-school use of Irish, motivation and proficiency in immersion and subject-only post-primary programmes. *International Journal of Bilingual Education and Bilingualism* 10, 428–453.

Rau, C. (2005) Literacy acquisition, assessment and achievement of year two students in total immersion in Māori programmes. *International Journal of Bilingual Education and Bilingualism* 8, 404–432.

Sagasta, M.P. (2003) Acquiring writing skills in a third language: The positive effects of bilingualism. *International Journal of Bilingualism* 7, 27–42.

Santiago, K., Lukas, J.F., Moyano, N., Lizasoain, L. and Joaristi, L. (2008) A longitudinal study of academic achievement in Spanish: the effect of linguistic models. *Language Culture and Curriculum* 2, 48–58.

Swain, M. and Johnson, R.K. (1997) Immersion education: A category within bilingual education. In R.K. Johnson and M. Swain (eds) *Immersion Education: International Perspectives* (pp. 1–16). Cambridge: Cambridge University Press.

Swain, M. and Lapkin, S. (1982) *Evaluating Bilingual Education: A Canadian Case Study.* Clevedon: Multilingual Matters.

Vila, F.X. (2008) Language-in-education policies in the Catalan language area. *Aila Review* 21, 31–48.

Zalbide, M. and Cenoz, J. (2008) Bilingual education in the Basque Autonomous Community: Achievements and challenges. *Language, Culture and Curriculum* 21, 5–20.

9 Assessment of Academic Performance: The Impact of No Child Left Behind Policies on Bilingual Education: A Ten Year Retrospective

Stephen J. Caldas

This chapter analyzes the American No Child Left Behind legislation in terms of its need, history, provisions for English Language Learners (ELLs) and consequences for ELLs and schools with large ELL populations. The chapter also considers possible forthcoming revisions to the reauthorized law, and speculates on how American ELLs will be educated in the future. Finally, the chapter answers the questions of whether the achievement gap with ELLs has narrowed, and whether ELLs were demonstrating higher academic outcomes in Mathematics and Reading in the period just prior to or after the implementation of NCLB.

Introduction

In 2001, the United States Congress reauthorized the Elementary and Secondary Education Act (ESEA) first passed in 1965, calling the new incarnation of the bill 'No Child Left Behind' (NCLB, 2001). This much more accountability orientated law, which represents the American federal government's official education policy, caused profound changes in how schools and students were assessed and evaluated. The massive NCLB legislation, almost 700 pages in length, has also caused a sea change effect in how American schools have been assessing and educating their bilingual and English Language Learner (ELL) students. Some of the effects of the bill have been intentional, others unintentional. Regardless of the intention of the law, it could be argued, as some have (see Menken, 2008), that NCLB has not only created official language education policy, but unofficial de facto language policy for American public schools as well. This chapter analyzes the bill in terms of its need, history, provisions for English Language Learners (ELLs) and consequences for ELLs and schools with large ELL populations. The chapter also considers possible forthcoming revisions to the law, and the possible future impact on how ELLs will be educated in the US. Finally, it tries to answer the questions of whether the achievement gap with ELLs has narrowed, and whether ELLs were demonstrating higher academic outcomes in Mathematics and Reading in the period just prior to, or after the implementation of NCLB.

Need for Language Education Policy

Under No Child Left Behind, schools are held accountable for boosting the achievement of all low-performing student subgroups, including ELLs. Many school districts have very high percentages of students classified as ELLs, such as Los Angeles, California, where fully one-third of the student body of the nation's second largest school system is composed of English learners (Llanos, 2010). Although ELLs in America speak literally hundreds of different languages, the large majority of ELL students in the US – fully 80% – are Hispanic/Latino (Pitoniak, 2009), indicating that Spanish is the most commonly spoken second language in American schools. Indeed, by 2010, fully 5.7% of the entire American population aged 5 and older spoke Spanish as a first language, but 'did not speak English very well' (Caldas & Caldas, in press). This equates to approximately 17.5 million native Spanish-speaking individuals in the US learning to speak English. This number is expected to mushroom. Fully 37% of all fourth-grade Hispanic students in American public schools are ELLs, as are 21% of all eighth-grade Hispanic students (Hemphill & Vanneman, 2011). Students in these two grades participate in the National Assessment of Educational Progress (the 'NAEP'), also known as 'the Nation's Report Card'. By contrast, ELLs comprise less than 1% of the White student population (Hemphill & Vanneman, 2011). NCLB mandates that all states receiving Title I federal funding participate in the NAEP. This requirement allows for national comparisons of Math and Reading scores between Hispanic ELLs, Hispanic non-ELLs, and Non-Hispanic Whites.[1] These sorts of critical comparisons will be made later in this chapter in an effort to determine what effects NCLB might be having on ELL achievement and on reducing the achievement gap in American public schools.

ELLs do indeed show significant achievement gaps on both state and national assessments, including the NAEP (Hemphill & Vanneman, 2011; Perkins-Gough, 2007; Snow & Biancarosa, 2003; White House Initiative on Educational Excellence for Hispanic Americans, 1999). Additionally, 31% of ELLs drop out of high school, compared to only 10% of children who speak

English at home (Short & Fitzsimmons, 2007). Thus, many education policy experts and others believe that steps must be taken to help ELLs succeed in American schools. However, an important question to be answered is whether the mandates in NCLB (or its soon to be reauthorized successor) actually help ELL underachievement. On this point, there is much debate, but as we will see shortly, the answer seems to be 'no'.

The History of ESEA and the Bilingual Education Act

In 1965, the US Congress passed the most comprehensive American federal education legislation in the country's history, named the 'Elementary and Secondary Education Act of 1965' (ESEA). This initiative was part of President Lyndon Baines Johnson's Great Society initiative to involve public schools in 'The War on Poverty' (Bankston & Caldas, 2009: 116–117). ESEA provided compensatory education funding to states and local education agencies (LEAs) to help educate disadvantaged students, the primary target of the legislation. The ESEA contained the stipulation that the act must be reauthorized by the US Congress every five years, and the bill has undergone significant revisions in each of its subsequent reauthorizations in 1968, 1974, 1978, 1984, 1988, 1994, and finally, in its most recent NCLB version, in 2001. At the time of this writing, the bill, which was scheduled to be reauthorized in 2007, was stuck in a long, politicized legislative process that had not yet resolved itself by mid-2013.

In 1968, the ESEA Act was amended and expanded to add a new component, Title VII, called 'The Bilingual Education Act' (1968). The BEA is the federal government's first formal recognition of the special needs of ELLs, then referred to as students with 'Limited English Speaking Ability' (LESA). The BEA provided competitive grants to LEAs to assist them in educating English learners in poverty. However, the BEA contained no mandates for educating ELLs, nor made any explicit reference to the creation of bilingual education programs. Initial federal funding under BEA amounted to only $7.5 million (Stewner-Manzanares, 1988).

An important U.S. Supreme Court case in 1974, *Lau v. Nichols*, would influence the direction of all subsequent federal legislation pertaining to the education of ELLs. The suit was brought by Chinese Americans against the San Francisco school district, arguing that the civil rights of the Chinese students who could not speak English were being violated because the school district was not providing the kind of additional assistance that this group needed to learn English and achieve in school. The case eventually wound up in the US Supreme Court, which ruled that the non-English-speaking Chinese students had the same rights to be afforded an opportunity to achieve as other students in the San Francisco school system. Being provided the same instruction as English proficient (EP) students, the Supreme Court ruled, was not adequate enough for these students, and violated the provisions of the Civil Rights Act of 1964, which prohibited discrimination based on color, creed or national origins. This case effectively linked minority language status with national origins, and thus culture.

When ESEA was reauthorized in 1974, it included a new act with direct implications for the education of ELLs, the Equal Education Opportunity Act (EEOA), as well as significant amendments to the BEA. As regards the EEOA, it prohibited LEAs from segregating students if such segregation would deny students educational opportunities based on race, color, sex or national origin. This provision would constrain districts from separating ELLs from the rest of the school population, based on the national origins provision of the act. As for the changes to the original 1968 BEA, the 1974 amendments included an explicit definition of a bilingual education program as including instruction in English and the child's native tongue. Also, under the amended BEA, funding for bilingual education programs was drastically increased to $68 million, a national clearinghouse on bilingual education research was established, the low-income restriction on federal spending for ELLs was removed, and bilingual program capacity building efforts in LEAs were stipulated in order to foster the creation of local language programs that would survive after federal funding ended (Stewner-Manzanares, 1988).

The 1978 reauthorization of ESEA amended the BEA to include a new definition for ELLs: Limited English Proficient (LEP). The LEP definition expanded upon the earlier LESA designation to include the notions not only of limited English speaking ability, but also of limited proficiency in reading, writing and understanding English to an extent that students would suffer in a classroom in which the language of instruction was English. Also, the 1978 amendments to the BEA now prohibited funding to programs designed solely to maintain native languages other than English (LOTE), and encouraged districts to transition 'LEPs' into regular education as soon as possible. Funding under the BEA of 1978 was increased to $135 million (Stewner-Manzanares, 1988).

The 1984 reauthorization of ESEA included several important amendments to the BEA (Title VII). These included a provision that allowed for up to 10% of Title VII funding to be used for 'special alternative instruction programs' which used only English instruction with 'LEPs'. Grants under the BEA were also awarded for developmental bilingual education programs that offered instruction in both English and the native language with the goal of developing proficiency in both languages. Grants could also be used for transitional bilingual education programs which emphasized using English and the ELL's native language to move the child in the direction of English language proficiency. Funding for the BEA of 1984, $139.4 million, was barely greater than the amount of funding authorized under the BEA Act of 1978, and a decrease of almost $30 million from 1980 (Stewner-Manzanares, 1988). The country was now under the presidency of the socially conservative

Republican, Ronald Reagan, and the BEA, as well as the entire ESEA Act, reflected to some extent the growing conservative educational ideology taking root in the country. The movement to the right, which demanded greater educational accountability, was ignited by the report 'A Nation at Risk' published in 1983 by the National Commission on Excellence in Education. The report lamented the deplorable condition of K-12 education in the United States, and ushered in the era of standardized curriculum and standardized testing (Bankston & Caldas, 2009).

Conservative ideas in education continued to gain traction throughout the decade of the 1980s. When ESEA was reauthorized in 1988, the BEA included several very important changes, including a provision that up to 25% of grant funding to districts could be used for 'special alternative instruction programs' (meaning they did not need to use native language instruction). The other 75% of funding had to be used for transitional bilingual education programs. There was now a three-year limit placed on how long most ELLs could remain in one of these specialized programs. The parents of ELLs now had to be provided with information in a language they understood advising them of their rights to refuse a Title VII program for their child. The gist of the changes to the BEA in this latest reauthorization could be interpreted as discouraging the bilingual development of ELLs.

In general, the 1988 amendments to the BEA included more flexibility to local districts in educating their ELLs. This was during a period of increasing immigration to the United States from Latin America and Asia, and a growing sense of urgency that ELLs needed to be transitioned to English-only classrooms as soon as possible. The educational reform movement, with a 'back to the basics' emphasis, stressed the need for more testing for students and greater accountability for teachers and schools. Ronald Reagan was completing his second term in office, and conservative, reactionary thought (reaction to 'excesses' of the 1960s and 1970s) had by the late 1980s thoroughly pervaded much educational thinking and policy making (Bankston & Caldas, 2009).

With the election of Democratic President Bill Clinton in 1992, there was a brief respite from the conservative wave sweeping the country. The 1994 reauthorization of ESEA, entitled 'Improving America's Schools Act of 1994' (IASA), included significant amendments to the BEA that reflected a new level of appreciation for bilingualism. The progressive tone of the bill has yet to be matched in federal education legislation. The preamble to Title VII now opened with the explicit acknowledgement that 'multilingual skills constitute an important national resource which deserves protection and development' (IASA, 1994, §7102). Moreover, the Act now acknowledged that developing 'bilingual skills and multicultural understanding' was an important goal of the Act, as well as developing, 'to the extent possible, the native language skills of such children and youth' (IASA, 1994, §7102).

This iteration of BEA actually gave preferences to programs that developed bilingual competencies over English language proficiency (Wiese & García, 1988). The 1994 BEA stated that a goal of the legislation was 'the preservation and maintenance of native languages,' referring specifically to Native American, Hawaiian, and Pacific Islander languages (IASA, 1994, §7122). In terms of the tension between assimilationist and multicultural philosophies of education, the 1994 BEA leaned more heavily toward the multicultural end of the spectrum (Wiese & García, 1988). It is not coincidental that the 1994 reauthorization of a more educationally progressive ESEA was signed by President Clinton. Clinton was a liberal democrat in a party that at the time provided a clear alternative to conservative Republican education ideas that were more narrowly focused on school accountability to the exclusion of more enriching educational experiences such as furthering bilingualism.

Paradoxically, also passed in 1994 was the Goals 2000 'Educate America' Act, which, with its emphasis on national, measurable outcomes, was in some ways inimical to the new-found appreciation for language diversity expressed in the 1994 IASA. Goals 2000 is the spiritual father of the much more prescriptive NCLB – an Act, which as we will see shortly, expresses little regard for the value of bilingualism. Goals 2000 set academic goals that were impossible to achieve, including the following: 'By the year 2000. . . *Every* [emphasis added] adult American will be literate and will possess the knowledge and skills necessary to compete in a global economy and exercise the rights and responsibilities of citizenship' (Goals 2000, 1994, §102). But at least the bill did not yet mandate the accomplishment of these impossible dreams. This was to come with NCLB.

The 2001 Reauthorization of ESEA: The No Child Left Behind Act of 2001

The 2001 reauthorization of ESEA, known as the 'No Child Left Behind Act of 2001' was signed into law on January 8, 2002, by the new, conservative Republican President George W. Bush. This new incarnation of ESEA represented the greatest change in American education policy since the bill first became law in 1965. Title VII, the Bilingual Education Act, was completely removed from the law, and with its removal all references to the term 'bilingual' were also eliminated. Title III, 'Language Instruction for Limited English Proficient and Immigrant Students' became the new federal policy for educating ELLs.

The preamble to the NCLB Act, which is only one sentence long, states the entire purpose of the new vision of federal education policy for the United States. This purpose is 'To close the achievement gap with accountability, flexibility, and choice, so that no child is left behind'. One of the explicit achievement gaps targeted for elimination was the gap between ELLs and non-ELLs.

NCLB'S General Orientation toward Educating ELLS

A surprisingly large part of the NCLB legislation deals either directly or indirectly with the education of ELLs (LEPs), although Title III was written expressly for the education of this student subpopulation. Title I, which includes provisions for 'Improving the Academic Achievement of the Disadvantaged,' also now pertains to ELLs, which the government has decided are at risk in the same way that children in poverty are at risk.

The number one purpose of Title III, which is entitled the 'English Language Acquisition, Language Enhancement, and Academic Achievement Act' is stated in Part A:

> To help ensure that children who are limited English proficient, including immigrant children and youth, attain English proficiency, develop high levels of academic attainment in English, and meet the same challenging State academic content and student academic achievement standards as all children are expected to meet. (NCLB, 2002, §3102)

Title III authorized the expenditure of $750 million in 2002 to carry out this act (§3001).

The thrust of every purpose delineated in the new Title III is toward the acquisition of English proficiency, followed by ELLs' meeting the same subject matter standards as other students, including English language arts. Title III contains no explicit reference to the terms 'bilingualism' or 'bilinguals' or 'multiculturalism,' unlike its 1994 predecessor. Rather, it uses the term 'Limited English Proficient' throughout to refer to students who are English learners, 'ELLs' (the preferred term in most education and linguistic circles). However, unlike some of the negative media coverage of NCLB, the act is not overtly or intentionally anti-bilingual, and indeed, expressly states in Part B of Title III that an intent of the law is to not only develop English proficiency, but, 'to the extent possible, proficiency in their [ELLs] native language' (§ 3211). Moreover, as regards the curricula used to accomplish these goals, NCLB states that federal funds can be used in 'developing and implementing programs to help children become proficient in English *and other languages* [emphasis added]' and 'acquiring or developing education technology or instruction materials for limited English proficient children including *materials in languages other than English* [emphasis added]' (§3212). The Act even mandates that in some programs the teacher must speak a language other than English proficiently if 'instruction in the program is in the native language as well as English' (§3214). NCLB even gives a nod to two-way dual language programs by defining a 'Language Instruction Program' in part as one that:

> 'may make instructional use of both English and a child's native language to enable the child to develop and attain English proficiency, and may include the participation of English proficient children if such course is designed to enable all participating children to become proficient in English and a second language. (§ 3303)

So, this author's reading of NCLB is not that it is necessarily against bilingualism. Rather, its main emphasis, as outlined in Title III of the Act, is the strong encouragement to states and districts to push hard for ELLs to first attain English language proficiency, and then continue to learn English (while advancing at the same pace as English-proficient students ('EPs') in the acquisition of content matter in other subjects). Although this was the government's plan, we will see below that the plan is not realistic and has had unintentional consequences in the education of ELLs.

As already noted, ELL students (LEPs) are classified under NCLB as students who are 'at-risk', suggesting that their language status (speaking a language other than English) is viewed almost exclusively as a handicap, with no redeeming benefits for the child. This macro perspective is in line with Ruíz's (1984) 'Language as a Problem' orientation, which is akin to seeing the child's language status as a learning disability, and not viewing the child's multilingualism as a resource to be developed and nurtured. So whereas the bill does allow for language instruction strategies that include use of the ELL's native tongue (as we will see below), almost the entire focus of all the bill's mandates is to push ELLs in the direction of English proficiency. This is an ironic position, because the field of linguistics has confirmed that proficiency in the L1 language is a predictor of how well one acquires the L2 language (Collier & Thomas, 2009; Cummins, 2000; Genesee, 1994; Genese et al., 2006; Goldenberg, 2008; Lindholm-Leary, 2001; Slavin & Cheung, 2005).

Trying to interpret, much less apply, the myriad of provisions contained in the NCLB Act as they pertain to ELLs is a difficult task (Rossell, 2005). The language is complex, legalistic, and in some cases, completely contradictory. As mentioned above, most of the provisions which pertain directly to ELLs are contained in Title III of the act. However, this subgroup of students (LEPs) is referenced throughout the entire voluminous law, so one would need to read all 670 pages of the Act (more than once, probably) to understand the federal government's entire position with regards to educating this subpopulation of students. As hard as the bill is to make sense of, the next section of this book chapter attempts to parse out specific NCLB provisions pertaining to ELLs.

Specific NLCB Mandates for ELLS

As a first step for states and school districts, NCLB requires that all states receiving funding under this Act identify those students who are ELLs. Most states do this initial assessment with a 'home language questionnaire' which asks the parents/guardians a few questions, including what is the primary language spoken by the child and the family. Students deemed to be potential ELLs based on the results of the home language questionnaire are typically given a state-developed English proficiency test based on their grade level, to establish their base level of English proficiency and make a determination of whether they are in fact not proficient in English. This is a problematic process, because, as Rossell (2005) notes, it is difficult for these tests 'to distinguish the difference between a student who does not know the answer and a student who does not know English' (p. 9). Once they are classified, NCLB requires that states annually assess ELLs using valid and reliable instruments to determine their progress toward attaining English proficiency (according to a standard that each state may determine individually) (NCLB, §1111). This information must be made public.

The parents of ELLs must be notified within 30 days after the beginning of the school year that their child was diagnosed as an ELL, or within two weeks of their initial diagnosis if they are admitted later in the year. The parents must also be told how their child was diagnosed, how he/she will be taught, and when the child is expected to be English proficient (or if a high school student, when they are expected to graduate, which for most ELLs is in the standard four years). The parent must be notified in a language he or she can understand (a provision that has resulted in an increased need for districts to hire interpreters). School districts must also draw up and implement plans to actively involve the parents of ELLs in the education of their children.

Language curriculum for ELLs

With regards to which language programs can be used to teach ELLs, in Title III of NCLB, the statute indicates that states and districts have:

> the flexibility to implement language instruction educational programs, based on scientifically based research on teaching limited English proficient children, that the agencies believe to be the most effective for teaching English. (§3102)

There is much debate in the education and linguistic communities about the best way to teach ELLs, ranging from those who argue for the transition of ELLs into English-only instruction as soon as possible to those who advocate developing the child's native language in tandem with his/her proficiency in English. Unlike the earlier reauthorization of the ESEA Act in 1994, NCLB does not explicitly acknowledge the benefits of an ELL's native language, seeming to put the federal government in the camp of those who emphasize moving the child quickly into English, without much regard for preserving his/her native tongue. The Act makes no direct reference to the commonly held knowledge in the linguistics community, based on much solid research (Collier & Thomas, 2009; Cummins, 2000; Genesee, 1994; Genesee *et al.*, 2006; Goldenberg, 2008; Lindholm-Leary, 2001; Slavin & Cheung, 2005), that the number of years of instruction in the child's L1 language is a key predictor of how quickly the child will advance academically in school in his/her L2 language (thus reducing the academic achievement gap, which is ostensibly the driving purpose of NCLB).

Two major reviews of hundreds of research studies on how ELLs learn, one of which was based on a very solid meta-analysis of valid quantitative research findings, concluded that teaching ELLs to read in their L1 language promotes their reading abilities in English (August & Shanahan, 2006; Genesee *et al.*, 2006). The language and tone of NCLB does not seem to recognize such findings, which have come to be regarded as relatively con-clusive in the linguistics research community. As noted above, NCLB does allude to dual language programs as a possible curricular option for which federal funds can be used. It does not, however, actively champion or encourage this approach, which according to some researchers is one of the best approaches for developing the native tongues of ELLs while at the same time actively fostering the learning of English (as well as developing fluency in a second language among EPs) (Collier & Thomas, 2009; Evans & Hornberger, 2005).

In short, it seems that the NCLB legislation was written in complete disregard of the huge and growing body of research that suggests that bilin-gually educated students ultimately perform better, not only than ELLs who get the 'English only' treatment, but, even by high school, than native English-speaking students (see Collier & Thomas, 2009 for an outstanding treatment of this subject). And while the provisions of NCLB and all previ-ous iterations of ESEA are primarily aimed at helping at-risk students, pro-grams like two-way dual language immersion have spillover benefits for higher socioeconomic EP students that include not only becoming fluent in a second language like Spanish or Chinese, but becoming multicultural as well (Baralis, 2010).

Setting standards for ELLs

Under NCLB, each state is required to establish Average Measurable Achievement Objectives (AMAO's) in designated subject areas for all sub-groups of students, including ELLs. Schools and districts are required to show Average Yearly Progress (AYP) toward the attainment of these AMAO's

(NCLB, §1111). By 2014, *all* students – ELLs included – are mandated to be proficient on their states' Reading and Math assessments, though many states have applied for and been granted an exemption from this provision provided they sign onto President Obama's Race to the Top initiatives.

For ELLs, AMAO's must be established in the areas of learning English (rate of improvement in acquiring English) and attaining English proficiency (percentage of ELLs who annually attain the standard of becoming 'English proficient' as defined by the state). However, ELLs must also demonstrate Average Yearly Progress on the Average Measurable Achievement Objectives set in the same content areas as EP students, such as math, language arts and science. Moreover, with some limited exceptions, ELLs must take these other assessments in English after having been in the United States for as little as one year (NCLB, §1111), even though research suggests that it takes 5 to 7 years to acquire the level of academic English to do well in school (Hakuta *et al.*, 2000).

With regards to learning English, districts are required to show that their ELL students are making Average Yearly Progress in acquiring English (as determined by steadily improving scores on English assessments), as well as acquiring proficiency in speaking, reading, writing and listening in English. Districts must show the number and percent of ELLs progressing in learning English and attaining English proficiency at the end of every academic year, and then track the progress of the newly English proficient students on state assessments in each of the next two years.

After ELLs have been in the US for at least one year, they must not only continue to demonstrate continual growth in learning English and advancing toward English proficiency, but they must also take all of the assessments that are required of English proficient students. Where tests are available, ELLs are allowed to take reading, language arts and subject area tests in their native language, as long as they are aligned with the content of the state's assessment instruments. (But they are not allowed to take these tests in a language other than English for more than three years, except with a possible two-year extension). However, ELLs must take the state's math assessment in English. Just as NCLB requires in relation to all other sub-groups of students, those districts and/or schools whose ELLs do not meet Average Yearly Progress standards for two consecutive years must develop school improvement plans. Those entities whose ELLs do not meet AYP standards for four consecutive years risk losing federal funding and/or having to fire staff deemed responsible for this 'failure' to achieve.

Contradiction and confusion

The NCLB requirement that districts must demonstrate that their subgroup of ELLs have made AYP goals in academic subjects, including English, just as English proficient students must do, has a built-in paradox.

The category of 'ELLs' is by definition a group of students who score low on measures of English. As Rossell (2005) has wryly noted,

> If you define a group by their low test scores, that group *must* have low test scores or someone has made a mistake. Once a LEP child's English test scores rise to the level defined by a state or local education authority (LEA) as the point at which they are English proficient (typically determined by a test tailored for limited English proficient children), they are no longer in the LEP group.... (p. 2)

The federal government, apparently recognizing this paradox, began allowing districts to keep FLEPs (Former Limited English Proficient students, known also as Fluent English Proficient [FEPs]) in the ELL category for up to two years after they have tested out, so that their typically higher test scores are reflected in the ELL subgroup. But even so, including FLEP students' higher scores is not enough to significantly boost the lower scores of the larger group of ELL students who still have not acquired English proficiency (Rossell, 2005). In short, the achievement gap between ELLs and non-ELLs can never be closed, as long as ELLs are defined by their low scores in English proficiency – the language in which most high stakes assessments are administered. Thus, districts with large ELL populations will always underperform, and ELLs can never be proficient on assessments administered in English – not in 2014, 2044 or 4044. NCLB insures, moreover, that we will always know exactly how large this gap is, because the Act requires annual program evaluations that compare ELL and EP student average scores on tests, including assessments that measure progress in reading, language arts and English proficiency.

In spite of the impossibility of ELLs ever being proficient on English assessments, NCLB still requires that ELL student test scores be aggregated with both special education students' and regular education students' scores in determining a school's overall AYP. This tenet of NCLB seems one of the greater injustices foisted upon school districts, and is one reason that the law is very likely to be changed when it is reauthorized. Schools and school districts with high percentages of ELLs will simply never be able to match the annual progress of districts with low percentages of ELLs on assessments administered in English.

In short, schools and school districts with large populations of ELLs are fighting an uphill battle to show the government mandated improvement on tests. However, at least NCLB does grant schools that are educating ELLs the eligibility to receive funding not only specifically designated for ELLs, but also allows funding to be used for ELLs that was formerly only to be used for economically disadvantaged students. Another positive mandate in NCLB is the requirement that school districts provide professional development for teachers in how to address the specific learning needs of the ELLs that they teach. NCLB also encourages the use of education technology (including the Internet) in furthering the instructional needs of ELLs (§3112).

NCLB and the Assessment of ELLS

So, we see that one very important consequence of NCLB for all students has been the ever greater importance placed on standardized testing and the use of test results for determining everything from grade promotion to high school graduation for students, and to whether schools are closed down and staff fired. The emphasis on test-driven accountability in the United States has probably had no greater impact on any other subgroup, except for perhaps special education students, than it has had on English learners. This disproportionate influence of NCLB on ELLs is attributable to the very real fact that in addition to testing for content area knowledge, all tests administered to ELLs in English (which are most of them) end up being English proficiency tests as well, whether or not this is the actual intent of the test.

There is an even larger issue, though, than the increased pressure on ELLs placed by the NCLB mandates necessitating frequent testing in the ELL's non-native, and by definition, non-proficient language. This larger issue is that NCLB testing mandates are creating ad hoc education language policy in the reality of everyday school practices (Menken, 2008; Zacher Pandya, 2011). Indeed, Shohamy (2001) noted that educational policies can be determined by studying testing policy. This is because, as Menken (2008) discovered in her research of practices on the ground in New York City schools, '... tests shape what content is taught in school, how it is taught, by whom it is taught, and in what language(s) it is taught' (p. 4). In short, tests dictate what happens in schools, and NCLB is built almost exclusively around test-driven accountability.

The reality that tests dictate much of what transpires in the school day of ELLs and their teachers is poignantly made in Zacher Pandya's (2011) ethnographic study of an elementary school in California where 70% of the student population was English learners, and 90% of the student body lived in poverty. The classroom teacher who Zacher Pandya shadowed was required to teach her 28 fourth-grade students (21 of whom were ELLs) the pre-packaged reading curriculum 'Open Court,' produced by SRA/McGraw-Hill. The program is scripted and highly regimented, and the observed teacher had to rush through material in order to stay on track and cover the required units in the academic school year. Over the course of the school year, the students were required to take six unit tests aligned with the Open Court curriculum as a requirement of the federal funding the school received through a Reading First grant. Students' benchmark scores on these skills tests were posted on a bulletin board for all to see, and were often openly discussed and analyzed in class, where individual student scores were publically compared with peers' scores. Every student was also required to take the California Standards Test (CST), on which no child in the observed class had yet scored as 'proficient'. California does not allow testing in a child's native language (US Department of Education, 2008). The CST, like most NCLB required state tests, was normed on native English speakers. As has been pointed out by psychometric experts, tests that are administered to groups for which they have not been designed and for whom they are not normed are inherently biased (AERA *et al.*, 1999). Every ELL in the school was required to annually take the California English Language Development Test (CELDT) in order to measure the child's level of English proficiency, and to make a determination about whether or not the child had at last become English proficient. In short, the observed fourth-grade students lurched from one test to another.

The children in Zacher Pandya's (2011) study were totally socialized into and co-opted by the testing culture of the school, as were students throughout this heavily tested California district. The ELLs in the school used the term 'benchmark' as a verb, as in 'I'm benchmarking this week' (p. 23). The children equated their abilities and 'place' in the educational hierarchy with the labels that came attached to their test scores, and Zacker Pradya described in depressingly sad detail how the system slowly eroded children's self-esteem. Zacher Pandya argued that the students had trouble decoding, much less comprehending, the wording used in the tests they took. Teaching was always oriented to the tests, and the tests themselves took away much instructional time from the well-meaning but harried teacher she observed.

NCLB does allow testing accommodations and modifications for ELLs, depending upon what is being assessed. Such accommodations might consist of extended time, having the test read aloud, and the use of glossaries and bilingual dictionaries. Plus, as noted above, NCLB allows ELLs to be tested in their native language for three, and with a waiver, for up to five years. New York State, for example, offers certain elementary grade content area tests and the state's high school Regents Exams (equivalent to graduation exit exams) in five languages. But not all states have language testing options like New York. In fact, only eleven states report offering at least one content area test in a language other than English (US Department of Education, 2008). Moreover, all ELLs across the US must still take English proficiency tests in the English language. Passing these and other high-stakes subject matter tests in English is often a requirement before a child can either move on to the next grade, and in most cases graduate from high school. On the face of it, this might seem like sound policy. The problem is, though, that ELLs are expected to graduate from high school in four years like everyone else, and if they do not, the school and district are penalized by having a lower published graduation rate.

In another telling study of how NCLB accountability was shaping practices at the secondary level, Menken (2006) interviewed dozens of educators in ten high schools, and the majority of ELL educators admitted that they 'taught to the test' (p. 526). Menken found that NCLB has changed school language policy by forcing educators to align their curriculum to the mandated high stakes tests that ELLs must take. Due to NCLB mandates, most of the NYC high schools in Menken's study teach more content in English (rather than the child's native tongue) to ELLs to help them pass the state's high stakes high school graduation exit exam. At least one NYC school in her study essentially doubled the amount of ESL instruction given to ELLs to help them pass the state (high school exit) Regents Exam, because the school wanted to ensure it would make Average Yearly Progress. Menken argues that as a consequence of NCLB's emphasis on passing tests, ESL pedagogy has moved away from teaching communicative oral competence in English, to teaching literary competence, which is what is needed to take tests. ESL classes are now more like English Language Arts classes for native English speakers, she says.

How has NCLB Changed the Landscape of Bilingual Education?

It depends upon one's point of view, and perhaps one's political and philosophical orientation, as to whether the effect of NCLB on ELLs has in general been positive or negative. Advocates for ELLs are likely to be happy that NCLB has resulted in many more districts receiving federal funding for ELLs than was the case prior to 2002 (Rossell, 2005). Individuals and organizations advocating for the rapid assimilation of ELLs into the English-speaking mainstream may be happy that the increased funding for ELLs is largely being used to increase proficiency and competency in English (and not further proficiency in the child's native language). For those who advocate the quick transition from instructing a child in his/her native language to English-only instruction, this curricular shift in teaching ELLs more English is probably well received.

Bilingual and multicultural education advocates, on the other hand, seem to be almost unanimous in their opposition to NCLB (as vocalized by the National Association for Bilingual Education, n.d.). Whereas the predecessor to NCLB, the Improving America's Schools Act of 1994, openly encouraged and validated the development of bilingualism, many have argued that NCLB seems to have had the effect of promoting the learning of English at all costs, including at the expense of the child's native tongue (Crawford, 2002; Evans & Hornberger, 2005; García, 2004; Menken, 2008). García (2004) contends that NCLB 'serves to further stigmatize, humiliate, and marginalize people who are not a part of the dominant culture' (p. 37). García goes on to emphasize that 'the authors of NCLB are smoke screening one of their motives for creating NCLB, which is to give states and local districts the freedom to do whatever it takes to drive up test scores, even if that means more Proposition 227-like measures and English-only policies' (p. 37). Proposition 227, passed in 1998, effectively mandated that ELLs in California state schools be instructed only in English (with some limited exceptions) (Zacher Pandya, 2011). García states that the heavy testing and accountability component of NCLB works against ELLs, because 'state mandated tests simply show what these students cannot do, because they are inherently based on a deficit model' (p. 37). García laments that NCLB serves to propagate dominant Anglo-American culture and values and keeps language minority children subservient and in the underclass. García concludes that 'In sum, NCLB, because it clearly seeks to maintain current present approaches to curriculum and assessment, is detrimental to English language learners and other ethnically diverse children' (p. 38).

As noted above, Zacher Padnya's (2011) findings provide evidence to substantiate some of García's concerns. Hispanic ELLs in the school she studied scored low on the many standardized tests that they took, and seemed to internalize the testing culture and the low scoring labels it assigned to them. A particularly heart-rending description of one fourth-grade ELL, 'Tara', who could not score above a 1 out of 10 on a Reading First Skills Assessment test tells how the child had to admit before her entire class, with downcast eyes: 'I got a one…I got a one' (p. 17). This kind of public humiliation of students runs counter to much sound pedagogy about how students learn, and seems anachronistic in the post Progressive Education Age, which was itself an early twentieth century movement against the rote learning and unpleasant educational surroundings which typified America during that period (Bankston & Caldas, 2009).

As discussed above, research has shown that developing a child's proficiency in his/her native tongue transfers over to his or her learning of English. The problem is that the academic benefits that come from developing a child's native tongue may not manifest themselves on assessments in English until after grade six – a point well outside the 2- to 4-year window in which schools must demonstrate Average Yearly Progress and accomplish their Average Measurable Achievement Objectives. This inconvenient truth has likely discouraged districts from expanding bilingual education programs like long-term transitional bilingual or dual language programs. This state of affairs might make anti-bilingual education advocates happy, but neglecting the development of a child's native tongue, according to most credible research, is not in the child's or a diverse society's best long-term interests. Although NCLB expressly states that educational entities can use whatever programs or curricula they see fit to educate ELLs, in reality the stipulations of AYP restrict the options available to schools and districts. It seems that 'teaching to the test' is the norm, as in order to make AYP, schools and districts are teaching ELLs the kinds of skills that high stakes tests measure. So, in this sense, NCLB has indeed created de facto language education policy in many schools and districts, even though on the face of it, the act promises flexibility and choice in choosing language curricula.

Ten Years Later, How Have ELLS Been Performing Academically?

This brings us to an important point in this discussion. Has the NCLB Act actually helped to reduce the achievement gap between ELLs and others, as it promised to do? And has the measurable achievement of ELLs improved more during the period that NCLB has been law than in the period prior to the passage of this educational accountability act?

Of all the tests that American students in K-12 schools must take, there is only one that allows the kinds of national and state-by-state longitudinal comparisons that would allow for an objective determination of whether subgroups of students are showing improvement over time. This test is the NAEP (National Assessment of Educational Progress), first administered in 1969, and is now taken in alternating years by a nationally representative sample of students, including ELLs, in all 50 states. The NAEP is administered by the National Center for Education Statistics within the US Department of Education.

NAEP specifically issues a report tracking the public school achievement levels of Hispanics (ELLs and non-ELLs) and Non-Hispanic White students over time on its fourth- and eighth-grade Reading and Mathematics assessments, which are administered to students *in English* in these grades (Hemphill & Vanneman, 2011). The NAEP first began disaggregating data by ELL status with the 1996 administration of its Mathematics test, and with the 1998 administration of its Reading test. It only reports data on Hispanic ELLs, as all other ELL subgroups are too small for these kinds of public analyses. Less than one percent of Non-Hispanic Whites who take the NAEP are classified as ELLs, so Non-Hispanic White ELLs are included in the broader subgroup of all Non-Hispanic Whites who take the test. The data in the NAEP achievement gap report are presented in such a manner that ELL and non-ELL achievement in Mathematics and Reading can be tracked and compared prior to and after the implementation of NCLB.

A couple of precautionary notes are in order here. First of all, because these tests are administered in English, and as ELLs are by definition not proficient in English, we can never expect ELLs to do better than non-ELLs on these sorts of assessments. What we can do, however, is use data from the NAEP to gauge any improvement ELLs might be showing on these tests (presumably due to changes in how ELLs are being educated), to compare differing rates of improvement in Math and Reading, and to compare the changing gaps over time between ELLs and non-ELLs. According to the logic of NCLB, the gaps between ELLs and non-ELLs should be decreasing on these NAEP assessments as a consequence of the law's educational mandates. An additional caution we must take into consideration in analyzing and comparing these test scores is that, although we are doing this in the context of changing federal policy (pre- and post NCLB), there are many factors that affect test scores: changing populations of students over time, changing practices in schools and homes that may have no connection to federal policy, and other extraneous factors.

NAEP Mathematics Results

The data presented in the Hemphill and Vanneman (2011) report on the NAEP achievement gaps between Hispanic ELLs, non-ELL Hispanics and Non-Hispanic Whites provides results through the 2009 administration of the NAEP. The report indicates that there were small, but statistically significant increases in the performance of Hispanic ELLs between the 2003 and 2009 administrations of the fourth- and eighth-grade Mathematics tests (p. 17). Whereas one cannot directly compare Hispanic ELLs with Non-Hispanic Whites, one can compare the achievement of Hispanic ELLs and non-ELL Hispanics on both the fourth- and eighth-grade NAEP Mathematics tests. Not surprisingly, non-ELL Hispanics scored much better than Hispanic ELLs on both the fourth- and eighth-grade Mathematics tests. However, the achievement gap between non-ELL Hispanic and Hispanic ELL fourth-graders actually increased between the 2003 and 2009 administrations of these tests, although the change was not statistically significant. Importantly, though, there was a statistically significant *increase* in the gap between non-ELL Hispanics and Hispanic ELLs on the eighth-grade Mathematics tests between 2003 and 2009. In short, the achievement gap on the Mathematics tests between Hispanic ELLs and non-ELL Hispanics did not decrease at the fourth-grade level, and actually increased significantly at the eighth-grade level.

I decided to make direct comparisons between student performance prior to and after the implementation of NCLB in 2002. I made these comparisons by calculating the absolute change in NAEP Mathematics scale scores for Hispanic ELLs, non-ELL Hispanics, and Non-Hispanic Whites in the period for which data on Hispanic ELL achievement first became available prior to the implementation of NCLB, which was 1996. As the Mathematics test was also given in 2003, I calculated the change in fourth- and eighth-grade Mathematics scores from 1996 to 2003—the pre-NCLB era (or as close to a pre-NCLB period as can be calculated). Then, I calculated the change in scale scores for each subgroup from 2003 to 2009, the NCLB policy era, and the last year for which data were available (see Table 9.1).

Table 9.1 [2]Change in NAEP scale score points in *Mathematics* before and after implementation of NCLB for public school Hispanic ELL, non-ELL Hispanic, and non-Hispanic white students: grades 4 and 8

	Hispanic ELLs	Non-ELL Hispanics	Non-Hispanic Whites
Grade 4			
1996–2003[3]	+13	+17	+13
2003–2009	+5*	+6*	+5*
Grade 8			
1996–2003[4]	+14	+9	+8
2003–2009	+2*	+8*	+5*

*2003 significantly different ($p < 0.05$) from 2009

As can be seen in Table 9.1, the Mathematics scale scores increased more during the pre-NCLB period (for all groups, in fact) than during the period since the implementation of NCLB. Looking at each student category and grade-level separately, we see some telling results. The increase for Hispanic ELLs was from two and one-half to seven times *greater* (at grade 4 and grade 8, respectively) during the period prior to NCLB's implementation compared to the period during which NCLB was the law of the land. In other words, the Mathematics achievement of Hispanic ELLs increased at a much faster rate under the more bilingual education-friendly 'Improving America's Schools Act of 1994' than it did under the much more accountability oriented NCLB Act of 2001. As for non-ELL Hispanics and Non-Hispanic Whites, the findings were similar: the Mathematics achievement of neither of these subgroups advanced as much during the NCLB era as they did during the period prior to the passage of NCLB. In other words, all these subgroups showed greater improvement on the NAEP Mathematics tests *prior* to the implementation of NCLB.

NAEP Reading Results

I followed the same procedures for determining change on the NAEP Reading tests pre- and post NCLB, although the span of years was not exactly the same due to the differing years that the Reading test was administered. The first year for which data on Hispanic ELLs was available on the NAEP Reading test was 1998. Thus, I looked at the period from 1998 to 2002 as the pre-NCLB era, and used the period from 2002 to 2009 as the NCLB era.

It is important to note that the Reading tests are likely even more dependent on a student's level of English proficiency than are the Mathematics tests. Thus, these comparisons are more sensitive to the effects of language policy, instructional strategies, and curricula. Again, using the Hemphill and Vanneman (2011) NAEP achievement gap report comparing 2002 with 2009, one can see in Table 9.2 that although there was a slight increase in fourth-grade Reading scores for Hispanic ELLs from 2002 to 2009, the increase was not statistically significant (p. 43).

On the other hand, there was actually a statistically significant *decrease* in eighth-grade Hispanic ELL Reading scores from 2002 to 2009. In short, Reading scores did not significantly increase for ELLs over the period of NCLB, and in fact significantly *decreased* on the eighth-grade test.

As regards the gap between non-ELL and ELL Hispanics, there was no statistically significant change in this substantial gap on the fourth-grade test between 2002 and 2009. However, there was actually a statistically significant *increase* in the gap between non-ELL and ELL Hispanic eighth-grade Reading scores between 2002 and 2009. So, gaps between Hispanic ELLs and non-ELLs not only did not narrow at either grade level, but actually *increased significantly* on the eighth-grade test.

Looking further, again, at a wider span, as I did above for Mathematics scores, Table 9.2 compares the growth of NAEP Reading scores in the pre-NCLB era with the growth in scores during the post-NCLB era among Hispanic ELLs, non-ELL Hispanics, and White fourth- and eighth-graders. In a similar pattern to what was observed with the change in fourth-grade Mathematics achievement pre- and post NCLB, Hispanic ELL growth on the fourth-grade Reading test *prior* to the implementation of NCLB was more than twice the growth rate in Reading scores observed during the NCLB era (Hemphill & Vanneman, 2011: 43). The more striking difference, though, was among eighth-grade Hispanic ELL Reading scores. Although there was an increase of seven points on the NAEP Reading test during the pre-NLCB period from 1998 to 2002, there was actually a statistically significant *decrease* of five points in Hispanic ELL Reading scores during the NCLB era from 2002 to 2009.

The differences in Reading achievement growth pre- and post-NCLB were not quite as great among non-ELL Hispanics and Non-Hispanic Whites. Nevertheless, for Non-Hispanic Whites, the growth in Reading scores prior

Table 9.2 [5] Change in NAEP scale score points in *Reading* before and after implementation of NCLB for public school Hispanic ELL, non-ELL Hispanic, and non-Hispanic white students: Grades 4 and 8

	Hispanic ELLs	Non-ELL Hispanics	Non-Hispanic Whites
Grade 4			
1998–2002[6]	+13	+1	+4
2002–2009	+6	+4*	+2*
Grade 8			
1998–2002[7]	+7	+6	+3
2002–2009	-5*	+4*	0

*2002 significantly different ($p < 0.05$) from 2009

to NCLB was twice the rate of growth of that observed during the NCLB era on the fourth-grade test, whereas Non-Hispanic Whites showed no growth at all on the eighth-grade reading test post-NCLB (though there was growth during the pre-NCLB era). Non-ELL Hispanics bucked the overall trend at the fourth-grade level, showing more growth post-NCLB than pre-NCLB. In summary, Hispanic ELLs showed much more growth pre-NCLB on both the fourth- and eighth-grade reading tests, and actually lost ground during the NCLB era at the eighth-grade level.

Summary of Hispanic ELL Academic Performance on NAEP

As noted above, we have to be careful making comparisons of ELLs on tests not normed for non-English proficient students. Nevertheless, we can draw some broad generalizations from this investigation on the only nation-wide assessment on which any sort of comparisons of this nature can be made. There is no evidence to suggest that the stated purpose of NCLB, which is to 'close the achievement gap,' is being accomplished based on NAEP data. In actuality, the NAEP data lend more support to the notion that if anything, the achievement gap between Hispanic ELLs and non-ELLs is growing at the eighth-grade level in both Mathematics and Reading. Moreover, it appears that ELLs were achieving at a faster rate in Reading and Mathematics prior to NCLB than after the passage of this accountability law. In summary, all the empirical evidence here suggests that the NLCB mandates for ELLs are not working, and, if anything, are having negative learning consequences for English learners.

Is it All that Bad?

There have been a few bright spots for ELLs in an otherwise drab gray NCLB landscape. For one, Hispanic achievement (including both ELLs and non-ELLs) has overall improved during the NCLB era on both the NAEP Mathematics and Reading tests at the fourth-grade level, and on the Mathematics test at the eighth-grade level. Non-ELL Hispanics also showed growth on the eighth-grade Reading test. But the growth in achievement has not been enough to close the gap with White students, and as we have seen in this study, all groups in general were showing more improvement on the NAEP prior to the implementation of NCLB. There are individual states that have fared better than others. Florida had closer scores between Hispanics and non-Hispanic Whites (less than half the national achievement gap) on the NAEP eighth-grade Reading test in 2009, making significant progress in reducing this gap over the period that NCLB has been law (Hemphill & Vanneman, 2011). This might be due to Florida's having mandated that all administrators and teachers who work with ELLs must take 60 hours of training, which according the Florida's chancellor, is 'focused on specific strategies about how best to teach someone learning the English language' (Sparks, 2011, June 23). Additionally, all English teachers in Florida have to receive 300 hours of ESL training.

Three years after NCLB became law, Capps *et al.* (2005) had speculated that, 'Since LEP students will be required to learn the same content and pass the same assessments as other students, NCLB could better integrate and align LEP students' classroom instruction with instruction provided to others' (p. 1). It is possible that ELLs are now receiving instruction more along the lines of what is being provided to non-ELLs. However, as we have seen, the education community has largely soured on the notion that ELLs should be taught the same way as EPs. Capps *et al.* further speculated that NCLB 'may alter language programs and produce an increased focus on rapid English acquisition' (pp. 1–2). There could well have been an increased focus on trying to help ELLs learn English, but based on the NAEP Reading results shared above, there is no empirical evidence that ELLs are in fact learning English at a faster rate under NCLB policy. One outcome does seem certain, though: ELLs are being tested to a degree never seen before. Perhaps the most conclusive evidence for the widespread disappointment with NCLB is the vast majority of states formally seeking waivers to suspend the punitive Average Yearly Progress requirements (US Department of Education, 2011a). Whereas some may lay the blame on states, districts and schools for not reaching the exalted standards for ELLs (and all other students) set by NCLB, a more reasoned and rational explanation is that the biggest problem is not with the schools or educators, but with an unworkable law.

The Next Reauthorization of ESEA

At the time of this writing, Congress is wrangling over the next required, long overdue reauthorization of ESEA. Although the outcome of Congress' deliberations remains uncertain, what seems crystal clear is that there has been widespread discontent with NCLB among educators who must labor under its punitive, utopian, and according to many experts, misguided and non-research-based mandates, especially as regards teaching ELLs (Menken, 2008). In 2010, President Barack Obama and the US Department of Education published 'A Blueprint for Reform' which emphasized his administration's priorities for the reauthorization of ESEA (US Department of Education, 2010). These included the goal, which actually seems as utopian as any in the 2002 version of the act, that all children will graduate from high school ready to go to college. This goal specifically references language minority children. The blueprint also states the government's intention to continue to fund and strengthen initiatives to benefit 'English learners' – the first time that this more current term will appear in a reauthorization of ESEA.

In some small ways the blueprint does take a slightly less harsh tone than NCLB, making statements such as 'State accountability systems will be asked to recognize progress and growth and reward success, rather than only identify failure' (p. 9). In a hint that the Obama administration wants to back away from Average Yearly Progress goals, the blueprint asserts that 'States, districts and schools will not just look at absolute performance and proficiency, but at individual student growth and school progress over time' (pp. 9–10).

However, the Blueprint includes what appear to be two new mandates for states regarding the education of ELLs. States would be required to:

- 'Establish new criteria to ensure consistent statewide identification of students as English Learners, and to determine eligibility, placement, and duration of programs and services, based on the state's valid and reliable English language proficiency assessment'; (p. 20)

and

- 'Implement a system to evaluate the effectiveness of language instruction educational programs, and to provide information on the achievement of subgroups of English Learners, to drive better decisions by school districts for program improvement, and to support districts in selecting effective programs'. (p. 20)

The Blueprint is clear that 'Schools that are not closing significant, persistent achievement gaps' (p. 10) fall into a category of 'challenge' schools where the administration and faculty could all be subject to being removed and the school closed. As noted in the discussion above, ELLs by definition will always score less well on assessments administered in English than will EP students, and under Obama's Blueprint, the testing requirements of NCLB would remain in place. Thus, there must always be a gap between ELLs and others (Rossell, 2005), and continued reliance on testing will continually remind us of this psychometric reality.

If it is any consolation for states and LEAs, the Blueprint at least indicates that funding will be available to develop and perfect these new required assessments of English language proficiency and assessments for ELLs. On another positive note, the Blueprint is more explicit about the type of educational programs for ELLs that federal funding can be used to support, including 'dual-language programs, transitional bilingual education, sheltered English immersion, newcomer programs for late-entrant English Learners, or other language instruction educational programs' (p. 20).

In October 2011, the Senate education committee completed a major, ten month re-write of NCLB that would eliminate the setting of annual performance goals, Average Yearly Progress, and in general return more authority over how schools are run to states and districts (Dillon, 2011). However, passage of this revised bill on the floor of the entire Senate without significant revisions was very uncertain. Moreover, action in the House of Representatives has been much slower and more piecemeal, with some speculation that the Republican controlled House did not want to see a reauthorized bill passed before the presidential election of 2012 that might have given Obama a major legislative victory (Dillon).

Relief?

Barack Obama, however, was not waiting for the passage of a reauthorized ESEA, and in September of 2011 authorized the Secretary of Education to issue waivers to states that would suspend Average Yearly Progress requirements in return for states agreeing to 'adopt college- and career-ready standards; link teacher, principal, and student data...and identify persistent achievement gaps within the State that need to be closed' (US Department of Education, 2011a). As an indicator of just how much discontent there is over NCLB's strict requirements, 41 states submitted requests to the Department of Education asking for these flexibility waivers (US Department of Education, 2011a). On February 9, 2012, the US Department of Education granted its first waivers to ten states, with more waivers expected to be granted throughout the year (Cavanagh & Klein, 2012). The future is not entirely hopeful though, as states are now beginning to wrestle with how to link ELL achievement with teacher and administrator evaluations (as is required by Obama's Race to the Top), a linkage that is very psychometrically questionable (Newton et al., 2010).

Concluding Thoughts

One conclusion that can be safely drawn about NCLB is that its provisions for ELLs are not really based on solid empirical research, but rather political expediency (Spolsky, 2009). Unfortunately, though, American public schools have no choice but to adhere to the stringent federal mandates under NCLB (or its successor) or risk losing federal funding, which amounted to over 100 billion dollars during the 2010–2011 school year (US Department of Education, 2011b).

It is striking how NCLB makes no reference to the importance of ELLs' (or any other students') maintaining or acquiring proficiency in languages other than English. For example, accurately identified ELLs almost by definition know another language fluently, yet there is no provision for states to help students maintain their native-like fluency in a non-English language. This is especially disheartening in light of research that indicates that the number of years of education one receives in one's L1 tongue is a good predictor of how well one will achieve in his/her L2 tongue—not to mention the benefits of multilingualism in a society as diverse as America's.

Finally, for those who just have to see a number, the evidence to support the major *raison d'être* of NCLB – the reduction of the achievement gap between subgroups like ELLs and others – is simply not there. There is actually more evidence to support the contrarian point of view that if anything, NCLB has exacerbated, not reduced this gap.

Notes

(1) The Department of Education tracks student achievement on its NAEP tests based on the five mutually exclusive racial/ethnic categories of White (non-Hispanic), Black (non-Hispanic), Hispanic, Asian/Pacific Islander, American Indian (including Alaska Native), and Unclassified. Hispanics may be of any race. The schools who participate in the NAEP provide the data on the racial/ethnic classification of the tested students. Though not an endorsement of the American government's racial classification schema, this chapter will use the racial/ethnic categories employed by the US Department of Education.
(2) Data were obtained from Hemphill, F.C. and Vanneman, A. (2011).
(3) Significant differences between 1996 and 2003 cannot be determined.
(4) Significant differences between 1996 and 2003 cannot be determined.
(5) Data were obtained from Hemphill, F.C. and Vanneman, A. (2011).
(6) Significant differences between 1998 and 2002 cannot be determined.
(7) Significant differences between 1998 and 2002 cannot be determined.

References

American Educational Research Association, American Psychological Association, & National Council on Measurement in Education. (1999) *Standards for Educational and Psychological Testing, 1999.* Washington, DC: American Educational Research Association Publications.

August, D. and Shanahan, T. (eds) (2006) *Developing Literacy in Second Language Learners: Report of the National Literacy Panel on Language Minority Children and Youth.* Mahwah, NJ: Lawrence Erlbaum.

Bankston, C.L. and Caldas, S.J. (2009) *Public Education – America's Civil Religion: A Social History.* New York: Teachers College Press.

Baralis, C.L. (2010) The long-term effects of a K-5 dual language program on middle school student academic achievement and biculturalism (doctoral dissertation). Retrieved from ProQuest. (3405271)

Bilingual Education Act, Pub. L. No. (90–247), 81 Stat. 816 (1968).

Bilingual Education Act, Pub. L. No. (93–380), 88 Stat. 503 (1974).

Bilingual Education Act, Pub. L. No. (95–561), 92 Stat. 2268 (1978).

Bilingual Education Act, Pub. L. No. (98–511), 98 Stat. 2370 (1984).

Bilingual Education Act, Pub. L. No. (100–297), 102 Stat. 279 (1988).

Bilingual Education Act, Pub L. No. (103–382), (1994).

Capps, R., Fix, M., Murray, J., Ost, J., Passel, J.S. and Heerewantoro, S. (2005) *The New Demography of America's Schools: Immigration and the No Child Left Behind Act.* Washington, DC: The Urban Institute. Retrieved at: http://www.urban.org/UploadedPDF/311230_new_demography.pdf

Caldas, S.J. and Caldas, S.V. (in press) Latinos and the demographic shift from minority to majority status. *Encyclopedia of Latino Issues Today.*

Cavanagh, S. and Klein, A. (2012, Feb. 9) Broad changes ahead as NCLB waivers roll out. Education Week. Retrieved at www.edweek.org.

Civil Rights Act of 1964, Pub. L. 88–352, 78.

Collier, V.P. and Thomas, W.P. (2009) *Educating English Learners for a Transformed World*. Albuquerque, NM: Fuente Press.

Cummins, J. (2000) *Language, Power and Pedagogy: Bilingual Children in the Crossfire*. Clevedon: Multilingual Matters.

Dillon, S. (2011, October 11) Bill would overhaul No Child Left Behind. *New York Times*. Retrieved from www.nytimes.com.

Elementary and Secondary Education Act of 1965, Pub. L. No. 89–10, 79.

Evans, B. and Hornberger, N. (2005) No child left behind: Repealing and unpeeling federal language education policy in the United States. *Language Policy* 4, 87–106.

García, F. (2004) Developing sociopolitical literacy. *Clearing House* 78 (1), 34–40.

Genesee, F. (ed.) (1994) *Educating Second Language Children: The Whole Child, the Whole Curriculum, the Whole Community*. Cambridge: Cambridge University Press.

Genesee, F., Lindholm-Leary, K., Saunders, B. and Christian, D. (2006) *Educating English Language Learners: A Synthesis of Research Evidence*. Cambridge: Cambridge University Press.

Goals 2000. Educate America Act, Pub. L. No. (103–227) (1994).

Goldenberg, C. (2008) Teaching English language learners: What the research does – and does not – say. *American Educator* 32 (2), 8–23, 42–44. Available at: http://www.aft.org/pdfs/americaneducator/summer2008/ae_summer08.pdf

Hakuta, K., Butler, Y.G. and Witt, D. (2000) *How Long Does it Take English Learners to Attain Proficiency?* Santa Barbara: University of California Linguistic Minority Research Institute.

Hemphill, F.C. and Vanneman, A. (2011) *Achievement Gaps: How Hispanic and White Students in Public Schools Perform in Mathematics and Reading on the National Assessment of Educational Progress* (NCES 2011–459). Washington, DC: National Center for Education Statistics, Institute of Education Sciences, U.S. Department of Education.

Improving America's Schools Act of 1994, Pub. L. No. (103–382) (1994).

Lau v. Nichols, 414 U.S. 563 (1974).

Llanos, C. (2010, May 21) More English-language learners at LAUSD, state test shows. *Daily News—Los Angeles*. Retrieved www.dailynews.com.

Menken, K. (2006) Teaching to the test: How No Child Left Behind impacts language policy, curriculum, and instruction for English language learners. *Bilingual Research Journal* 30 (2), 521–546.

Menken, K. (2008) *English Learners Left Behind: Standardized Testing as Language Policy*. Clevedon: Multilingual Matters.

National Association for Bilingual Education (n.d.) *Educational equity and excellence for ELLs*. Retrieved from: http://www.nabe.org/advocacy.html

National Commission on Excellence in Education (1983) *A Nation at Risk: The Imperative for Educational Reform*. Washington, DC: US Department of Education.

Newton, X., Darling-Hammond, L., Haertel, E. and Thomas, E. (2010) Value-added modeling of teacher effectiveness: An exploration of stability across models and contexts. *Educational Policy Analysis Archives* 18 (23). Retrieved from http://epaa.asu.edu/ojs/article/view/810

No Child Left Behind Act of 2001, Pub. L. No. 107–110, 115 Stat. 1425 (2002).

Pitoniak, M.J., Young, J.W., Martiniello, M., King, T.C., Buteux, A. and Ginsburgh M. (2009) *Guidelines for the Assessment of English language Learners*. Princeton, NJ: Educational Testing Service.

Ruíz, R. (1984) Orientations in language planning. *NABE Journal* 8 (2), 15–34.

Shohamy, E. (2001) *The Power of Tests: A Critical Perspective on the Uses of Language Tests*. London: Longman/Pearson Education.

Short, D. and Fitzsimmons, S. (2007) *Double the Work: Challenges and Solutions to Acquiring Language and Academic Literacy for Adolescent English Language Learners – A report to the Carnegie Corporation of New York*. Washington, DC: Alliance for Excellent Education.

Slavin, R. and Cheung, A. (2005) A synthesis of research on language of reading instruction for English Language Learners. *Review of Educational Research 75*, 247–281.

Sparks, S.D. (2011, June 23) Study finds gaps remain large for Hispanic students. *Education Week* 30 (36). Retrieved at www.edweek.org.

Spolsky, B. (2009) *Language Management.* Cambridge: Cambridge University Press.

Stewner-Manzanares, G. (1988) *The Bilingual Education Act: Twenty years later, (6), Occasional papers in bilingual education*. Washington, DC: The National Clearinghouse for Bilingual Education.

Twyman, T., Ketterlin-Geller, L.R., McCoy, J.D. and Tindal, G. (2003) Effects of concept-based instruction on an English language learner in a rural school: A descriptive case study. *Bilingual Research Journal* 27 (2) 259–274.

US Department of Education (2008) *Biennial Report to Congress on the Implementation of the Title III State Formula Grant Program, School Years 2004–06*. Washington, DC: Office of English Language Acquisition, Language Enhancement, and Academic Achievement for Limited English Proficient Students.

US Department of Education (2009) *National Assessment of Educational Progress (NAEP), various years, 1996–2009 Mathematics assessments*. Washington, DC: Institute of Education Sciences, National Center for Education Statistics.

US Department of Education (2010) *ESEA Blueprint for Reform.* Washington, D.C. Office of Planning, Evaluation and Policy Development,

US Department of Education (2011a) *ESEA flexibility.* Retrieved from http://www.ed.gov/esea/flexibility

US Department of Education (2011b) *The Federal role in Education.* Retrieved from http://www2.ed.gov/about/overview/fed/role.html.

Wiese, A. and García, E.E. (1988) The Bilingual Education Act: Language minority students and equal educational opportunity. *Bilingual Research Journal* 22, 1–18.

Zacher-Pandya, J. (2011) *Overtested: How high-stakes Accountability Fails English Language Learners.* New York: Teachers College Press.

Definitions of Alphabetisms

AMAO	Average Measurable Achievement Objectives
AYP	Average Yearly Progress
BEA	Bilingual Education Act
ELL	English Language Learner (formerly known as LEPs)
EP	English Proficient student
ESEA	Elementary Secondary Education Act
FLEP	Former Limited English Proficient student
IASA	Improving America's Schools Act
LEA	Local Education Agency
LEP	Limited English Proficient student
LESA	student with Limited English Speaking Ability (no longer used to refer to ELLs)
NCLB	No Child Left Behind Act
NEAP	National Assessment of Education Progress

10 Summary of Issues Surrounding the Assessment of Bilinguals and the Way Forward to Solutions

Virginia C. Mueller Gathercole

The chapters in this volume have raised several issues key to understanding the patterns of language acquisition and use in bilinguals and how these impact on assessment, whether of language itself or of abilities that go beyond language. The issues raised have highlighted the following:

Bilingual children and adults differ in important ways from monolingual children and adults. They differ in the timing of development of vocabulary and syntax, as well as in their knowledge of the two languages (Chapters 2, 5). For a complete picture of language knowledge in bilinguals, then, when possible, assessments should examine the bilingual's performance in both languages; and assessments should be developed that are normed against similar populations with similar experience with the language(s) in question (Chapter 2).

Bilingual performance may differ in subtle ways from that of monolinguals. Even adults who have grown up as bilinguals and who appear to perform within the norms for each of their languages may have grammars that differ in subtle ways from those of monolinguals and even from those of other bilingual groups (Chapter 5). This is more likely to be the case in relation to the minority language of the community than the majority language (Chapters 2, 5, 8). The differences in performance may be observable in one realm or with one measure (e.g. reaction times) even if they are not observable in another (Chapter 6); they may be influenced by the fact that many bilingual speakers learn their languages in the context of sociolinguistic flux (Chapter 4); and they may interact in complex ways with socioeconomic status (Chapters 3, 5).

At times practitioners – e.g. speech therapists or teachers – may not themselves know the first language of the bilingual child or adult they are working with, and may not have access to materials or assessment measures in that language, but may need to assess linguistic, cognitive, or academic abilities nevertheless. One goal might be to try to find language-neutral means of testing language abilities (Chapter 3), a goal that gains greater importance as our world continues to shrink. Another might be for a teacher to draw on resources available through the internet to help the L2 language-learning child in the classroom bridge from the L1 to the L2 and to use the L1 in assessing academic abilities until the child's L2 is established (Chapter 7; see also Chapter 8).

One question that frequently arises is whether the acquisition of several languages and use of more than one language in the classroom might adversely affect children's performance in academic realms. This question seems to be answered resoundingly in the negative on a number of counts. First, the performance of children growing up in bilingual settings in a number of areas of the world, such as the Basque country, demonstrates that they perform on tests of academic abilities at a level that is equivalent to (or better than) that of their peers in other settings (Chapter 8). Second, an examination of academic performance of children growing up before and after the implementation of the No Child Left Behind legislation in the United States, an act that has often been interpreted as dictating English-only classrooms, reveals that, in fact, bilingual children in general performed better before the implementation of such policies than after (Chapter 9).

All of these considerations together lead to the undeniable conclusion that the means used for testing bilingual children – whether to gain a full picture of their linguistic abilities or knowledge or to assess nonlinguistic performance – are in drastic need of revision. The chapters in the second, companion volume, *Solutions for the Assessment of Bilinguals*, take up this theme and propose some creative and innovative solutions to many of these issues.

Index of Tests and Measures

Index of Languages

Index of Terms

Quintessentials for General Dental Practitioners Series

in 50 volumes

Editor-in-Chief: Professor Nairn H F Wilson

General Dentistry, Editor: Nairn Wilson

Implantology in General Dental Practice	available
Culturally Sensitive Oral Healthcare	available
Dental Erosion	available
Managing Orofacial Pain in Practice	Autumn 2006
Dental Bleaching	Autumn 2006
Special Care Dentistry	Autumn 2006
Infection Control for the Dental Team	Spring 2007
Therapeutics and Medical Emergencies in the Everyday Clinical Practice of Dentistry	Spring 2007

Oral Surgery and Oral Medicine, Editor: John G Meechan

Practical Dental Local Anaesthesia	available
Practical Oral Medicine	available
Practical Conscious Sedation	available
Minor Oral Surgery in Dental Practice	available

Imaging, Editor: Keith Horner

Interpreting Dental Radiographs	available
Panoramic Radiology	available
Twenty-first Century Dental Imaging	Autumn 2006

Periodontology, Editor: Iain L C Chapple

Understanding Periodontal Diseases: Assessment and Diagnostic Procedures in Practice	available
Decision-Making for the Periodontal Team	available
Successful Periodontal Therapy – A Non-Surgical Approach	available
Periodontal Management of Children, Adolescents and Young Adults	available
Periodontal Medicine: A Window on the Body	available

Endodontics, Editor: John M Whitworth

Rational Root Canal Treatment in Practice	available
Managing Endodontic Failure in Practice	available
Restoring Endodontically Treated Teeth	Autumn 2006

Prosthodontics, Editor: P Finbarr Allen

Teeth for Life for Older Adults	available
Complete Dentures – from Planning to Problem Solving	available
Removable Partial Dentures	available
Fixed Prosthodontics in Dental Practice	available
Occlusion: A Theoretical and Team Approach	Autumn 2006

Operative Dentistry, Editor: Paul A Brunton

Decision-Making in Operative Dentistry	available
Aesthetic Dentistry	available
Communicating in Dental Practice	available
Indirect Restorations	Summer 2006
Choosing and Using Dental Materials	Autumn 2006

Paediatric Dentistry/Orthodontics, Editor: Marie Therese Hosey

Child Taming: How to Cope with Children in Dental Practice	available
Paediatric Cariology	available
Treatment Planning for the Developing Dentition	available
Managing Dental Trauma in Practice	available

General Dentistry and Practice Management, Editor: Raj Rattan

The Business of Dentistry	available
Risk Management	available
Quality Matters: From Clinical Care to Customer Service	Summer 2006
Practice Management for the Dental Team	Autumn 2006
Dental Practice Design	Autumn 2006
Handling Complaint in Dental Practice	Autumn 2006

Dental Team, Editor: Mabel Slater

Team Players in Dentistry	Autumn 2006

Quintessence Publishing Co. Ltd., London